Migraine in Childhood

Related titles:

Epilepsies of Childhood, 2nd edition (O'Donohoe)
Mechanism and Management of Headache, 4th edition (Lance)
Manual Therapy for Chronic Headache (Edeling)
The Child with Febrile Seizures (Wallace) (John Wright imprint)

Migraine in Childhood

and other non-epileptic paroxysmal disorders

Edited by **Judith M. Hockaday** MD Cantab., FRCP
Consultant Paediatric Neurologist, Department of Paediatrics, John Radcliffe Hospital, Oxford;
Honorary Clinical Lecturer, University of Oxford

Butterworths

London   Boston   Singapore   Sydney   Toronto   Wellington

First published 1988

© Butterworth & Co. (Publishers) Ltd, 1988

British Library Cataloguing in Publication Data

Migraine in childhood: and other non-epileptic
  paroxysmal disorders.
  1. Children. Migraine
  I. Hockaday, Judith M.
  618.92′857

  ISBN 0-407-01590-6

Library of Congress Cataloging in Publication Data

Migraine in childhood: and other non-epileptic
  paroxysmal disorders
  edited by Judith M. Hockaday.
    p.   cm.
  Bibliography: p.
  Includes index.
  ISBN 0-407-01590-6
  1. Migraine in children.
  I. Hockaday, Judith M.
  [DNLM: 1. Migraine – in infancy &
  childhood.   WL 344 M6358]
  RJ496.M54M54 1989
  618.92′857 – dc 19
  DNLM/DLC
  for Library of Congress   88-19465

Photoset by Butterworths Litho Preparation Department
Printed and bound in Great Britain at the University Press, Cambridge

Foreword

Migraine was described as long ago as three thousand years before Christ. Since that time there have been numerous publications concerning the disorder in adults, and even two hundred years ago cases of migraine with an early onset during childhood were discussed. However, the first investigations on children with migraine were not reported until the third and fourth decades of the present century. At that time paediatric textbooks contained only a few lines about chronic headaches, and migraine, in childhood. No information was given about the frequency of migraine or about special characteristics in children, and nothing was mentioned about what happens when the migraine child grows up.

Professor Bo Vahlquist in Uppsala was one of the few who at that time took an interest in these problems and made studies in childhood migraine. In 1955, he prompted me to start two investigations in this area, a study of the prevalence of migraine at school age and a longitudinal study. In the first study of about 9000 schoolchildren of ages 7–15 years it was found that 1.4% of the 7-year-old children experienced migraine, whereas by the age of 15 this prevalence had increased to 5.3%. Other investigators have since found similar or sometimes higher figures. In the second study 73 children with more pronounced migraine were followed up and reviewed four times over a 30-year period. During puberty and young adult life 62% had remissions for 2 years or longer, but in many migraine returned, and in 1985, after 30 years' follow-up, 53% still had migraine. A study of the next generation of these 73 migraine subjects showed that the girls, now grown up and mothers, had more children of their own with suspected migraine than the boys.

During the past three decades a gratifying increase in the interest in childhood migraine and associated paroxysmal disorders has been observed, in particular regarding the epidemiology and pharmacological treatment. A number of studies have now been carried out concerning prophylactic and attack-arresting drugs in children, similar to those used in adults, and some of them have shown good effects. However, the most important preventive measure in childhood is still thorough information to the child, the parents and the teachers regarding the migraine complaint. Of interest in this field is the psychological approach to the management of migraine and tension headache that has emerged in recent years. In children, as in adults, tension headache often follows the migraine attack or alternates with it. Studies of the effects of relaxation training and biofeedback treatment are in progress in several countries and these forms of therapy seem to show promising results. In childhood different variants of migraine can occur, including equivalents of migraine, and other paroxysmal disorders without headache, and interest in these problems has also increased during recent years.

Nowadays, migraine features more frequently in the paediatric textbooks than 30 years ago, and both paediatricians and neurologists devote much more attention to this common complaint. The International Headache Society, for example, has recently formed a study group focused on paediatric headaches. In 1984, an eminent book on migraine and other headaches in childhood was published by Dr Charles Barlow in Boston (Barlow, 1984): now the present book will be another good contribution to the increasing knowledge about childhood migraine and associated disorders.

Dr Judith M. Hockaday is a paediatric neurologist with well-known and broad knowledge of migraine in childhood. The experts she has collected as contributors to this book will together with Dr Hockaday be a good guarantee of its great value to neurologists, paediatricians and general practitioners.

Bo Bille
Department of Paediatrics,
University Hospital,
Uppsala

Preface and acknowledgements

It's just a headache, it's nothing really.

I heard this said, many years ago, by a paediatrician, to the mother of a young boy with severe migraine. His sleep was disturbed, school absence was increasing, and the visual aura was frightening to the child and alarming to all observers. I decided then that one day I would write a book to show that migraine in children is not 'just a headache'.

Dr Charles Whitty first introduced me to migraine about the time of the first migraine symposium at The Institute of Neurology, Queen Square, London, in 1966. I am grateful to him for the opportunities which followed to study the disorder. I am also very grateful to friends and colleagues in many countries, who have encouraged my interest, and referred many fascinating cases.

I would like to thank my secretary, Mrs Jean K. Barclay, for her friendship and support over many years of work together. I thank her also for her very considerable secretarial skills, and for her qualities of patience, tact and understanding in helping look after my patients.

I am aware of the ambiguities in this book. Migraine is indefinable. There is a central core of knowledge about it that is clear and generally acceptable. Then there are widening circles of uncertainty, which include fascinating clinical phenomena, about which there is much disagreement. My intention has been to give at least some attention to all these, however remote their relationship to migraine might appear. The approach is therefore overinclusive rather than underinclusive. This in turn leads to some overlaps, and some contradictions, as my co-authors and I express our individual opinions. I think these are inevitable until we know more about migraine and the other non-epileptic paroxysmal disorders discussed.

I am grateful to my co-authors for doing what I asked them to do, however arbitrary their chapter outline might appear. They have covered wider aspects than I could have achieved unaided, and have helped enormously in presenting the wide bibliography I was hoping for.

I am also most grateful to John Wilson for his 'personal' view – the result of many years' experience of ordinary, and rare and difficult forms of migraine, and of much thought about the uncertainties of the subject.

Finally, I would like to thank Bo Bille for first drawing the outlines of the subject of migraine in childhood. They still hold, and only the details are being added. I was delighted that he agreed to write a foreword to this volume.

Judith Hockaday
April 1988

Contributors

Thierry W. Deonna MD
Assistant Professor, Neuropediatric Unit, CHUV, Lausanne, Switzerland

Ian Forsythe MD, FRCP (Ed.)
Consultant Paediatrician, The General Infirmary at Leeds

Judith M. Hockaday MD Cantab., FRCP
Consultant Paediatric Neurologist, Department of Paediatrics, John Radcliffe Hospital, Oxford;
Honorary Clinical Lecturer, University of Oxford

Gwilym Hosking MRCP, DCH
Consultant Paediatric Neurologist, Ryegate Children's Centre and Children's Hospital, Sheffield

Richard W. Newton MD, MRCP, DCH
Consultant Paediatric Neurologist, Royal Manchester Children's Hospital and Booth Hall Children's
Hospital, Manchester

R. C. Peatfield MD, MRCP
Senior Registrar in Neurology, The General Infirmary at Leeds

John Wilson MB BS, PhD, FRCP
Consultant Neurologist, Hospital for Sick Children, Great Ormond Street, London

Dewey K. Ziegler MD
Professor of Neurology, Kansas University College of Health Sciences, Kansas City

Contents

Abbreviations

ACM	acute confusional migraine
AH	alternating hemiplegia
BAM	basilar artery migraine
BPT	benign paroxysmal torticollis of infancy
BPV	benign paroxysmal vertigo of childhood
CSF	cerebrospinal fluid
CT	computerized tomography
EEG	electroencephalogram
IPS	intermittent photic stimulation
MAO	monoamine oxidase
PCR	photoconvulsive response
PMi	pronounced migraine (Bille, 1962)
RAP	recurrent abdominal pain
RAST	radioallergosorbent test
REM	rapid eye movement
SAH	subarachnoid haemorrhage
TGA	transient global amnesia

Glossary

Many terms used in discussing migraine are used differently by different authors. In this volume usage is as follows:

abdominal migraine	an equivalent of migraine with prominent abdominal pain
abortive migraine	neurological aura symptoms occurring independently of headache
classical migraine	migraine with neurological aura
common migraine	migraine without neurological aura
complicated migraine	neurological deficit prolonged beyond duration of headache
equivalent of migraine	migraine without headache
migraine accompagnée	migraine headache accompanied by non-visual sensory or motor deficits or speech disturbance (term in use in European literature)
migraine dissociée	neurological aura symptoms occurring independently of headache
variant of migraine	an unusual form, which however fulfills usual diagnostic criteria for migraine

Migraine: a personal view

John Wilson

T'were better a fertile error, than a sterile truth. (Anon.)

There is a widespread belief that the practice of paediatrics is merely general medicine scaled down, and that children are mini-adults. This view is misleading and ignores not only differences in tempo of disease, for example infections, but also in manifestations of diseases sharing a common aetiology with conditions seen in adults. This is clearly seen in the study of childhood migraine, where paediatricians are as interested in the non-neurological as in the neurological manifestations of disease. Of course, as expanded in subsequent chapters, much of the symptomatology of migraine as described in adults is instantly recognizable in children. However, there is also a wide acceptance, at least among paediatricians, that other phenomena peculiar to childhood, for example so-called cyclical vomiting, limb pains and the periodic syndrome, are part of the more complex symptomatology of migraine in early life. Paediatricians are thus more ready to accept a widening of the concept of migraine than general neurologists who prefer a more cranial orientation. Some of the resulting disagreement arises from a failure to distinguish between the constraints imposed by a strict definition of a name, 'migraine', and the flexibility necessary in *describing* a disease, with its inherent biological variation. The one may have value in identifying a number of patients who have common characteristics, rigidly defined, to try to ensure homogeneity, to serve as a core group in the search for a discriminatory laboratory test, or in the elucidation of aetiology, pathogenesis and treatment. It is not essential, and indeed is not desirable that the descriptive process should be bound by narrow and rigid definition, since this may shackle exploration of significant phenomenology.

Of course, in the absence of a specific and characteristic test for migraine, it is impossible to prove that phenomena are migrainous. Moreover, every new episode, however typical, can bring a new problem of diagnosis for the clinician, because, with rare exceptions, symptoms and signs are not completely specific. This is especially true in children, but fortunately, after several attacks, most patients and their parents have sufficient confidence in their diagnosis, as well as more than a modicum of stoicism, to wait for the resolution of the latest attack unaided by outside consultation. However, the mimicry of pyogenic meningitis, with severe headache, neck stiffness and fever, or of an acute abdomen, will mean inevitably that some children will require lumbar puncture or laparotomy to resolve diagnostic uncertainty.

It is also appropriate for me to declare a life-long interest in migraine, first of all unknowingly as a child when all but the briefest of visits to the cinema were followed by a 'sick headache', and later with the morbid insight of a medical student. I count myself fortunate to have escaped (I hope) the perils of calomel poisoning, the result of the well-intentioned but utterly misguided recommendation of an elderly medical practitioner for what was almost certainly abdominal migraine. Well-remembered gnawing epigastric-central abdominal pain, ill-defined tenderness and altered bowel habit resolved in spite of, rather than because of, this perilous treatment. Now, as a parent myself, I can well understand the overweening anxiety of my own parents at the sight of a pale, drawn face and dark encircled eyes in an age and in an area where tuberculosis was rampant. I knew the unpleasant quality of the growing pains which Apley later recognized as a symptom associated with abdominal migraine and which is perhaps a juvenile equivalent of Ekbom's syndrome. Having married a migraineur I have enlarged my spectrum of closely observed symptomatology and have had ample opportunities (four) to ponder the genetic implications of this malady.

Whereas the temptation to absorb a miscellany of benign symptoms and signs into the pleomorphism of migraine is almost irresistible, and is inimical to scientific detachment, being a fellow sufferer confers a certain sympathetic insight.

But how wide is the spectrum? If the prevalence of migraine defined rigorously is of the order of 30% in the adult population, there is at least a one in three chance that any symptom or sign, neurological or otherwise, will coexist with migraine coincidentally, in children as in adults. In the absence of a discriminatory laboratory test, it is impossible on clinical and epidemiological grounds alone to identify a common pathogenesis between, for example, benign paroxysmal vertigo, periodic syndrome, abdominal migraine and classical migraine. Endeavours to show that symptoms and signs of different syndromes coexist more frequently than can be due to chance are complicated by the difficulty of enumerating a *predisposition* to migraine as opposed to migraine recognized and identified clinically. In a syndrome where exogenous factors including stress, food, temperature and trauma are important, clinical expression will reflect the chance interplay of (several) exogenous influences and an innate diathesis. For this reason, estimates of the frequency of a predisposition to migraine must be considered unattainable at present, but it is likely to be considerably greater than the frequency of migraine diagnosed clinically. It is also possible that the study of those uncommon individuals who deny *ever* having a headache even as a response to trauma, temperature or infection, may be equally informative, and provide a useful control group for biochemical as well as clinical studies.

In acknowledging the obstacles to a comprehensive nosology of migraine, nevertheless I believe the following childhood syndromes are migrainous in nature: benign paroxysmal torticollis, benign paroxysmal vertigo, abdominal migraine and the periodic syndrome. The latter is a condition characterized by episodic malaise, sometimes with fever. Attacks last hours or days and are often associated with abdominal pain, pallor, anorexia, nausea or vomiting, constipation or loose, clay-coloured stools resembling those of coeliac disease. In between attacks the child is well, and attacks may be heralded by exuberant well-being and voracious appetite. As mentioned above, I also include painful and restless legs as part of the childhood phenomenology of migraine, and believe that there is an increased frequency of epistaxis and earache usually with flushing of the pinna and sometimes with reddening of the drum in children with migraine as usually defined.

In a study with colleagues (Egger *et al.*, 1983) on the possible role of dietary factors in the pathogenesis of severe childhood migraine, an array of associated symptoms and signs such as abdominal pain, flatulence, loose stools, conduct disorder, aching limbs, rhinitis, aphthous ulcers, vaginal discharge, asthma and eczema responded with the headaches to a hypoallergenic diet which suggests that very diverse constitutional features are part of a highly complex syndrome. This study also provided the first double-blind validation of the association between diet and migraine. The fact that many placebo responders were excluded during a preliminary open trial was a strength of this study, not a weakness. In our series of patients, the role of precipitants such as physical and psychological stress, hunger and physical trauma were all recognized, but interestingly, once the source(s) of dietary sensitivity were excluded, other factors no longer served as precipitants. This may indicate that there is a threshold for attacks, and although diet itself may be sufficient to exceed the threshold in particularly vulnerable patients, for many others attacks only occur when other factors summate or multiply the dietary effect.

One of the other intriguing features in our study was the frequency of seizures in the whole group, selected for the frequency of headaches and resistance to conventional treatment and not because of the occurrence of seizures. Seizures remitted with headaches, and this encourages a more systematic study of the possible role of diet in childhood epilepsy.

Epileptic fits and migraine occur together more frequently than can be due to chance in children as in adults. Certain clinical features, such as focality and transient weakness, are common to both, and there is considerable overlap between the two. In a recent investigation, yet to be published, a hypoallergenic diet was more likely to be successful in producing a seizure remission in children who also have migraine than in those who had not; in the latter group, dietary manoeuvres were almost uniformly unsuccessful in our hands. It is unclear, however, if migraine can act as one of the many precipitants to seizures in a susceptible child, or are seizures an integral part of the migraine process?

Neuraxial vulnerability in migraine

The role of physical factors such as trauma in evoking a migraine attack is well recognized in children, and the migrainous significance of supposed 'concussion' after trivial head trauma has been emphasized. Given the cerebrovascular/ depolarizing instability that this implies, it is arguable that migraineurs may be particularly vulnerable to various potentially encephalopathic insults, metabolic, toxic and infective. However, evidence such as comparative data on the relative frequencies of, for example, encephalitis complicating the exanthemata in migrainous and non-migrainous children is lacking.

The possibility that deviant behaviour of cranial blood vessels is representative of a more widespread vascular instability also deserves consideration. In addition to thermographically demonstrable abnormalities of cutaneous perfusion of the face and scalp between recognizable migrainous episodes, spontaneous bruising elsewhere has been reported. Do perfusion changes – with reduction as well as increase – occur elsewhere? Does this confer a special hazard of myocardial ischaemia in patients whose arteries are already narrowed by atheroma? Is this related to increased platelet adhesiveness? Do peptic ulcers represent mucosal infarcts, and explain the association between peptic ulceration and migraine?

In speculating thus it is difficult to provide an explanation for the obviously different distribution of pathology and of much of the focal symptomatology of migraine. However, in the research priorities imposed by the present state of knowledge, anatomical considerations are of less importance than more dynamic aspects of pathogenesis.

The paediatric setting of this fascinating syndrome provides a particularly valuable opportunity for the study of a disease which is remarkable as much for its enmeshed relationship between psychiatry and organic neurology as for its enigmatic symptomatology.

Chapter 1

Definitions, clinical features, and diagnosis of childhood migraine

Judith M. Hockaday

. . . a highly prevalent, acutely morbid, and often incapacitating disorder. (Linet and Stewart, 1984)

Headache, including migraine, is an important symptom in childhood both because it is extremely common and because it may be symptomatic of serious disease. Bille (1962) found a prevalence of 59% in 8993 schoolchildren aged 7–15 years, and others (Waters, 1974a; Deubner, 1977; Collin et al., 1985) reported even higher figures (Table 1.1). It is such a common symptom, even in childhood, that it must usually be of little clinical significance, and indeed most (81%) children experiencing headache in Bille's study did so very seldom. However, Sillanpåå (1983a) found that 28% of children aged 14 years had headache at least once a month, and Moss and Waters (1974) observed that 27% of girls aged 10–16 years had consulted their doctor at some time because of headache. In another study the same investigators found that 27% of boys and girls who experienced headaches had severe attacks at least once monthly (Small and Waters, 1974). While organic causes are uncommon, some are very important, for example, Jerrett (1979)

Table 1.1 The prevalence of headache, and migraine, in children of school age, figures derived from published data

Author	Subjects	Age (yr)	Headache (%)	Frequent non-migraine (%)	Migraine (%)*
Vahlquist (1955)	1236	10–12		13.3	4.5
Bille (1962)	4440 boys	7–15	58	5.9	3.3
	4553 girls		59	7.7	4.4
Dalsgaard-Nielsen et al. (1970)	1075 boys	7–18			6.8
	952 girls				7.5
Waters (1974a)	367 boys	10–16	85		9.0
	410 girls		93		12
Deubner (1977)	213 boys	10–15	74		16
	211 girls		82		22
Sparks (1978)	12543 boys	10–18			3.4
	3242 girls				2.5
Sillanpåå (1983a)	2921	7	37		2.7
	2921	14	69		10.6
Collin et al. (1985)	306	9–12	76		

* Ascertained on different criteria.

reported two children with cerebral tumour among 200 patients of all ages presenting with headaches to a general practice list of 2550 patients in a 2-year period, and Honig and Charney (1982) found that when brain tumour in childhood does cause headache, then it is highly likely to be the first symptom (80% of their series).

If acute headache occurring with constitutional upset or trauma is excluded, then the majority of headache syndromes in childhood are recurrent and unexplained in the sense that no abnormal physical signs indicating an organic aetiology can be found. Migraine falls into this category. Indeed, together with tension headache, it probably accounts for the great majority of unexplained recurrent headaches in childhood.

Definition

Uncertainties about definition, and the absence of a marker or test for migraine, can make diagnosis difficult at any age. In children the difficulty is increased by early presentation. Understandably, and correctly, children tend to be brought for medical consultation early in the course of a headache disorder, before a recurring pattern with continuing good health between attacks (typical of migraine) can bring reassurance that the disorder is benign. Again, although given time, children can provide adequate accounts of their symptoms, this is only according to their intellectual development and experience, so that the history may well be limited by failure to remember early headache, or head trauma, or to recognize and be able to describe phenomena such as sensory disturbance, diplopia or vertigo. Children may also be slow to recognize or complain of change such as increasingly severe headache, or the onset of new symptoms such as unsteadiness. Evaluation of a headache disorder, and the diagnosis of migraine in children thus requires careful observations repeated over a period of time (for further discussion see below).

Despite considerable recent advances in the understanding of pathogenesis, migraine is still a clinically defined disorder and it is over- or underdiagnosed according to which, and how many, of its many characteristic features are regarded as relevant. The many attempts at definition reflect the uncertainties. There is also the difficulty that migraine is probably a heterogeneous disorder. Leviton (1984) wrote: 'What clinicians call migraine probably is a number of disorders each with its own metabolic or physiological characteristic. It is highly unlikely that all children labelled as migraine sufferers have the same deficiency or aberration.' Linet and Stewart (1984) came to similar conclusions in their excellent epidemiological review, referring to the need to recognize the heterogeneity of migraine and the existence of distinct aetiological subtypes.

In general, headache is regarded as migraine if it is paroxysmal and associated with at least two of the following three features: lateralized pain, nausea with or without vomiting, and focal neurological aura – these being found to be the characteristics most significantly associated with headache disorders diagnosed as migraine by experienced clinical neurologists (Waters, 1973). It is very difficult to identify migraine as a syndrome by epidemiological study and the idea that migraine is merely at one end of a spectrum of headache disorders has long been suggested (Waters, 1973; Kurtz et al., 1984).

In diagnosis of migraine in children the early approach first described by Vahlquist (1955), and followed by Bille (1962), has been widely accepted. Bille diagnosed migraine when headaches were paroxysmal, separated by symptom-free intervals and associated with at least two of these four features: one-sided pain; nausea; visual aura (or equivalent); family history of migraine in parents or siblings. Prensky and Sommer (1979) suggested a definition which took into account some of the special aspects of childhood migraine; they proposed association between headache and at least three of these six features: abdominal pain, nausea or vomiting; headache confined to one side; a throbbing or pulsatile quality of the pain; complete relief after a brief period of rest; an aura either visual, sensory or motor; a history of migraine headaches in one or more members of the immediate family. Congdon and Forsythe (1979) proposed a less strict modification of Vahlquist's approach, requiring three of these four features: an aura; nausea; vomiting; a family history; they observed that had they used the stricter criteria of Vahlquist (1955) and Bille (1962) some of their cases would have been excluded from diagnosis for some years (the stated difference in methodology, however, is not clear). At follow-up of at least 4 years (between 10 and 15 years in most), four children with classical migraine had died, one during a convulsion, one from drowning, and two from brain tumours which were diagnosed because of increasing headache frequency in one, and recurrence of symptoms after four headache-free years in the other.

Other suggestions for criterion diagnosis are more complex. For example, Baier and Doose (1985) listed six 'strong' associated symptoms (vomiting, scintillating scotoma, diplopia, pareses, paraesthesiae, aphasia) and six 'weak' symptoms (nausea, vertigo, photophobia, dread of noise, onset on awakening, relief after sleep) valued as only half as significant. In contrast, Kurtz *et al.* (1984) used an association between recurrent sick headache (headache with anorexia or nausea) and either vomiting or specific visual disturbance as evidence that headache was migrainous. For epidemiological purposes this is almost certainly as valid as more sophisticated methodology.

Criterion diagnosis of this sort is necessary for epidemiological study, and to enable case collection and comparison. However, it is unsatisfactory for clinical practice, where adherence to the above methods of ascertainment may not exclude symptomatic migraine nor necessarily include classical migraine (if scintillating scotoma is the only associated feature, as can be the case). There are other difficulties, too, in applying this approach in childhood when prostration, nausea, repeated vomiting and abdominal discomfort may overshadow the complaint of headache, and when the classical focal neurological aura (visual scintillations, scotomata) may well be infrequent, as has been found in some studies (Hockaday, 1979; Barlow, 1984). There can thus be risks in applying the usual principles in childhood groups.

Tal *et al.* (1984) 'tested' criterion diagnosis in migraine, and concluded that although 'migraine is not a very "secure" diagnosis in childhood' there was 'no proof that its use carries a significant danger of missing more important diagnoses'. They diagnosed 115 children as having migraine and studied outcome according to whether diagnosis had been positive (fulfilling two of Bille's four criteria) or possible (fulfilling only one of Bille's four criteria). The mean duration of follow-up was 5.4 years. Unfortunately 42 patients were lost to follow-up. However, the findings in those who were followed were reassuring in that only one change in diagnosis (from migraine to sinusitis), and no important new diagnosis, emerged in 36 'positive', or in 28 'possible' cases. It would have been interesting to learn how often a history of migraine in the family was the sole criterion in the 'possible' group. The diagnoses in five cases of hemiplegic migraine were also secure. (The outcome in four children originally diagnosed as abdominal migraine was far from satisfactory however, in that important new diagnoses emerged in two cases, see Chapter 4.) Tal *et al.* (1984) also found that provided Bille's criteria were followed, children with brain tumour who had a history of headaches and vomiting for more than 3 months and who had no abnormal neurological findings and who were thus 'candidates for a mistaken diagnosis of migraine' would not have been mistakenly so diagnosed. On their customary practice, cases where the history was shorter would not have been candidates for the diagnosis of migraine, 3 months or less being 'a period too short for a reliable diagnosis of migraine'. This is an interesting and helpful study but there are difficulties. The failure to obtain follow-up reports of 42 of the 115 migraine children must leave doubt about their outcome, and, despite the reassuring findings in the brain tumour group, many would be uneasy at the implication that a history of migraine in a family member (one of Bille's four criteria) should influence clinical diagnosis in a child with headache and vomiting. These and other aspects of differential diagnosis are discussed more fully below.

On this background, use of criterion diagnosis for migraine carries risks which are unacceptable in clinical practice. An alternative, simpler and clinically safer approach which avoids the difficulties was described by Hockaday (1982), who proposed that in childhood recurrent paroxysmal headache should be accepted as migraine provided there is return to full normal health both mental and physical between attacks, and that other causes of headache have been excluded. The method demands a period of observation in order to establish that normal health is indeed maintained between attacks. Diagnosis is thus both by *exclusion* and *longitudinal*. A family history of migraine is not used in diagnosis. In a series of 122 children who were diagnosed on this basis as having migraine (Hockaday, 1979) it was found that two or three of the three chief features of migraine were indeed present in 61%, thus validating the diagnosis in ordinary terms, and at least one was present in a further 33%. Only 6% lacked all three features commonly held to characterize migraine (unilateral headache, nausea/vomiting, aura). It was recognized and accepted that in these the distinction between common migraine (migraine without aura) and tension or psychosomatic headache was unclear and indeed that both might coexist.

There are a number of reasons why the presence or absence of a *family history of migraine is not used*. The most obvious is that such a history is often unreliable: where exact clinical diagnosis is uncertain, that by hearsay is even more so. Again, headache prevalence figures are in general so high that an account of familial headache must very often be by chance alone. Finally, there is still uncertainty about the nature of the genetic component in migraine. In a large epidemiological study, Waters (1971) found that although migraine was reported more often in near family members of migraine subjects than in families of subjects with non-migraine headaches, or those without headache of any sort, the differences did not reach statistical significance. Ziegler *et al.* (1975) and Lucas (1977) concluded from twin studies that the genetic component in migraine is much less than generally accepted, and while an epidemiological study in children by Deubner (1977) found evidence of a familial pattern, again this did not reach statistical significance. The topic is well reviewed by Goldstein and Chen (1982) and by Linet and Stewart (1984), and also see Chapter 2. One important reason for difficulty and uncertainty has of course been the use of the presence of a family history of migraine in case ascertainment by many authors. Another is the likelihood that while a subtype of 'genetic' migraine very probably exists, evidence for it is obscured in studies which merge all forms of migraine into a single heterogeneous group. Finally, the existence of migraine in near family members does not necessarily indicate that it is genetically determined: near family members often share the same environment.

Barlow (1984) also does not attempt diagnosis by criterion. In his volume on headache and migraine in children in which he describes his personal series of 300 cases, he states that 'personal criteria . . . are consistent with those used by other authors and especially those of Prensky (1976) and Friedman *et al.* (1962a) but *in the final analysis they represent a personal clinical impression*' [author's italics].

Conclusion

At this point it is concluded that identification of migraine by different 'sets' of positive criteria, such as those first propounded by Vahlquist in 1955, is acceptable and necessary for epidemiological and other study purposes. None is acceptable for clinical use. Many are marred by inclusion of a history of migraine in the family. None, with the exception of that of Tal *et al.* (1984), includes any suggestion for the necessary period of observation and none in present use excludes symptomatic migraine. Until migraine can be identified by some investigation or marker, it should remain within the area of headache problems in general, with diagnosis by exclusion of other causes.

The nature of the migraine attack

The most striking and indeed the only essential feature of the migraine attack is that it is paroxysmal. The attack is a sometimes most profound disturbance, fully reversible (except in rare instances), which occurs in otherwise normal subjects – as far as can be ascertained at the present time. It usually consists of headache associated with many other non-headache symptoms (common migraine), and may be marked by an aura of symptoms and signs of focal neurological disturbance (classical migraine). It is usual to consider hemiplegic migraine, basilar artery migraine, and ophthalmoplegic migraine, and some other rare presentations, as special forms or variants: these are discussed in Chapter 3. It is unlikely that there are any important differences between migraine in children, and in adults. Nearly all series have shown a slight preponderance of boys, attacks are often very brief and very frequent, and non-cranial (vegetative) symptoms may be prominent, but these are probably inessential variations.

The headache

Much has been written about the distribution and quality of the headache in migraine. However, such details are not always easily available in children nor are they very helpful in diagnosis. The headache of migraine may well have a throbbing quality and thus merit the description of 'vascular-type' headache; but so also do many headaches due to brain tumour (Raskin and Appenzeller, 1980). Head pain in migraine may be unilateral but is often not – indeed it is most often bifrontal. Some regard migraine as an unlikely diagnosis if headache is mild, but many patients, both children and adults, maintain that their headache is not severe and that either the aura or the non-cranial symptoms of the attack are more disturbing. In general fewer than 50% of children experience severe head pain. In addition, much has been written about the intellectual, personality and class characteristics of migraine subjects. There is no proper evidence that these help in definition, nor do various studies show much uniformity. Nor is there agreement on an apparent association between migraine and other disorders such as travel sickness and somnambulism, or on its relationships with so-called periodic syndromes (see Chapter 4), epilepsy (see Chapter 7), and allergies (see Chapter 8).

The characteristic that defines the headache of migraine more than any of the above is its periodicity or pattern of recurrence; this is reflected by the opening of the definition by the World Federation of Neurology Research Group on Migraine and Headache (1969): 'A familial disorder characterized by recurrent attacks of headache, widely variable in intensity, frequency and duration . . . (special) characteristics are not necessarily present in each attack or in each patient.' It would be inappropriate here to detail the observations on intensity, frequency, duration and distribution reported in many studies, varying widely, and largely depending on the populations from which case series have been drawn – specialist clinics clearly seeing a selected profile of the disorder, very different from community studies which in turn however usually lack clinical detail.

The most useful review in childhood is still that by Bille (1962), who described his findings in 347 children with migraine in a large population (8993) of schoolchildren, and gave additional clinical detail on those (73) with pronounced migraine, the PMi group (having severe attacks, lasting at least 1 hour, once a month or more). Others, including Waters (1974a), Sparks (1978), Hockaday (1979) and Congdon and Forsythe (1979) in the UK, and Prensky and Sommer (1979) and Barlow (1984) in the USA, report more recent observations, both in community and specialist clinic studies. The findings in the study by Congdon and Forsythe (1979) are typical. These authors recorded their experience of 300 children with migraine who had been followed for at least 4 years, most for 10–15 years. There were 177 boys and 123 girls with migraine, starting before age 5 in 102, between ages 6 and 10 in 166, and between ages 11 and 14 in 32. The most likely migraine frequency was once monthly (34%), but headaches could recur as often as two to three times a week (in 20% of the series; this high frequency was also noted by Bille, 1962). The headache was described as frontal in 65%, unilateral in only 31% and bitemporal in 4%. It was most likely to occur at any time of day (in 54%) but was quite often likeliest before rising (17%) and only rarely occurred typically at night (in 4%). Average duration was most often brief, between 0.5 h and 5 h in 61%, and only rarely exceeded 24 h (4%). The brevity of attacks in children was also noted by Bille (1962), Waters (1974a) and Sparks (1978). Prensky and Sommer (1979) noted that headache was bifrontal in 56% of their series, and Barlow (1984) noted hemicranial distribution in only 22%. Severity of headache is very difficult to judge, depending on many variables both within and outside the child. In young children estimation of headache severity is not possible, and overt measures of distress (such as need to lie down, or crying) may be due primarily to other symptoms. In older children Sparks (1978) observed that about 15% of boys and girls aged 10–18 reported they had mild attacks, while 46% of girls and 37% of boys had severe attacks – again this might reflect severity of non-headache symptoms. Small and Waters (1974) found very severe (or worse!) headache reported by 18% of boys and 12% of girls with migraine, and quite severe headache reported by a further 22% of boys and 35% of girls.

The amount of school absence caused by headache may be taken as another measure of its frequency and severity. Estimates of absence due to headache including migraine vary widely. A retrospective study in the UK found that over 50% of children with migraine in independent schools had missed school because of headache in the previous year (Sparks, 1978). Collin *et al.* (1985) did not find that headache was an important cause of school absence: it accounted for only approximately 1% of all school missed. In this study, in a school population with headache prevalence varying from 76% to 94% according to age, only 3.7% of children were absent because of headache during a two-term observation period. Of the 26 children absent because of headache, only three were away on more than one occasion, and of the 34 headache absences recorded, 85% were for one day or less. In a large community study Kurtz *et al.* (1984) found that 16-year-olds with sick headaches had markedly more school absence than their headache-free peers, but this was due to a very wide variety of reasons, and absence specifically caused by headache was not presented separately. Passchier and Orlebeke (1985) carried out a detailed community study of headache and stress in 2300 school pupils aged 10–17 years, and found 88% (of 2181 analysed) had headaches in the previous year. Less than half of these (42%) had missed school because of headache, and absence was almost always occasional (median 1–2 days); the median total of absence in the previous year was still only 3 days in the subgroup with weekly headaches (J. Passchier, 1985, personal communication).

Non-headache symptoms

Headache is only one part of the migraine attack. Associated malaise, gastrointestinal symptoms and other disturbances of vegetative (autonomic) function are common. They include changes in vasomotor control, with tachycardia, pallor or flushing, alterations of mood, appetite, thirst, sleep, fluid balance and temperature, and yawning, hiccupping and feelings of extracranial discomfort (and, rarely, pain) which is typically abdominal but may occur elsewhere. The volume by Sacks (1970) gives good descriptions of the variety of the non-headache symptoms. Klee (1968) also discusses them in detail, and his tabulation (Table 1.2, derived from his data) shows them occurring before, during and after the headache phase: 20% of his series had attacks of migraine starting before the age of 10 years. The possible mechanisms underlying these disturbances of hypothalamic function in migraine are well discussed by Herberg (1975).

The most typical of the non-headache symptoms of migraine are gastrointestinal. In the series reported by Congdon and Forsythe (1979), 94% of 300 children had nausea and vomiting, 5% had nausea only and 1% had vomiting without nausea – indeed to have one or the other was a necessary diagnostic criterion. Community studies have reported nausea in 50% of cases (Sparks, 1978), 79.5% (Bille, 1962), and in a series of 122 children ascertained by exclusion of other diagnoses, and not by criterion (Hockaday, 1979), nausea with or without vomiting was still a very typical feature, occurring in 75%. In Barlow's study (1984), where diagnosis was also clinical and not strictly criterion based, 62% of 300 children experienced nausea and vomiting, and a further 12% had anorexia alone. Claims that gastrointestinal disturbances are more likely or more prominent in children are often made, but this is difficult to substantiate from published data, and gastrointestinal symptoms can be prostrating at any age. The prominence of abdominal discomfort or pain as a vegetative symptom in the migraine attack varies

Table 1.2 Symptoms from vegetative nervous system before, during and after migraine headache (figures taken with permission from Klee (1968) Table 5, III, p. 56)

Nature of symptom	Total	Relationship to migraine headache		
		Before	During	After
At least one symptom	98	14	98	20
Nausea	88	2	88	0
Vomiting	90	2	90	0
Diarrhoea	18	2	18	0
Frequency of micturition	56	6	42	12
Sweating	50	0	50	2
Thirst	48	4	32	12
Oedema	42	2	42	0
Shivering, feeling cold	36	0	36	2
Lacrimation	22	0	22	0
Feeling of warmth, flushing	18	8	18	0
Diverse symptoms	14	0	14	0

Figures represent percentage values, derived from 50 patients.

considerably from one author to another. It is well described both in children and in adults by Sacks (1970) and severe abdominal pain was observed during the attacks in 5 of 29 children with basilar artery migraine (Hockaday, 1979). In contrast, neither Klee (1968) nor Herberg (1975) describe abdominal discomfort or pain in otherwise very wide series of observations (see Chapter 4).

The aura

Migraine is regarded as 'classical' or 'common' according to the presence or absence of an aura of focal neurological disturbance. This is most typically visual, and some authors restrict use of the term 'classical migraine' to attacks where the aura consists of flashing lights (photopsia), patchy scotomata, or an enlarging scotoma with scintillating zigzag edges (likened to the layout of the walls of a medieval fortress and called therefore fortification spectra, or teichopsia). At the present time it is usual in the UK to follow the terminology of the World Federation of Neurology (1969) which describes classical migraine as attacks in which headache is preceded or accompanied by transient focal neurological phenomena, e.g. visual, sensory or speech disturbances. The separation between classical and common migraine may not be essential. Most patients who experience classical attacks also have common migraine with the headache and non-headache symptoms being identical in both. The separation may be artificial and possibly only a matter of degree of severity of the underlying neurological disturbance (for fuller discussion see Wilkinson, 1986). The distinction becomes important for diagnosis only if it is made so, i.e. if the occurrence of an aura is regarded as a prerequisite for diagnosis. However, delineation of the aura is extremely important for management, differential diagnosis, and treatment.

Sacks (1970) discusses the variety, complexity and multiplicity of aura symptoms, and states: 'it is rare to encounter a single symptom in the course of a migraine aura'. Some, such as the scintillating scotoma, are fairly obvious, others such as brief sensory phenomena, less so; and some psychic phenomena, such as hallucinations and perceptual distortions of vision or sound, are likely to be described, by children particularly, only after persistent questioning. Hachinski *et al.* (1973) describe the visual symptoms observed in 41% of 244 children with migraine with excellent detail (see Chapter 7). In Bille's (1962) series visual aura was described by 50% of children with migraine, this figure rising to 70% in the PMi group. It lasted between 1 min and 30 min, most often about 5 min. Sensory disturbances, typically paraesthesiae, were also common (26% in the PMi group). Disorders of body image and distortions of size, shape and movement of objects (metamorphopsia) were described also, although these were rare (4 out of 347 cases). Congdon and Forsythe (1979) noted that an aura occurred prior to the attack in 107, at the time of headache in nine, and within 5 min of onset of headache in two, in 118 children with classical migraine. The aura was visual in 94: blurring of vision, 33; diplopia, 14; field loss, four; 'everything goes small', five; stars or flashes of light, 17; coloured circles, nine; spots, ten; and 'everything goes red', two. Three of the group had limb weakness, two numbness, and one 'stiffness' in a hand. In addition these authors listed some visceral symptoms occurring in 18 children prior to headache as auras: in other series these would be likely to be included as non-headache symptoms (see above), rather than as 'focal neurological disturbance'. In the study by Prensky and Sommer (1979) from a paediatric neurology clinic, visual aura was noted in 32% of cases, and sensory motor or speech problems in another 10.7%. In a series of 122 children also from a paediatric neurology clinic, diagnosed by exclusion of other cause for headache, Hockaday (1979) observed visual aura (teichopsia, unformed hallucinations, scotomata) in only 9% and unilateral sensory (with or without motor) disturbance in only two children, but other focal neurological disturbance was common – observed in 59 (48%) of the series overall. The majority of neurological symptoms were those suggesting basilar artery migraine, which was diagnosed positively (two or more specific symptoms) in 29, and possibly (one suggestive symptom such as vertigo or ataxia) in a further 18. This high proportion of basilar artery migraine (24% and possibly a further 15%) exceeds the incidence in most studies. Thus Barlow (1984) observed that only seven of his 300 cases of childhood migraine had migraine of basilar type, judged on a 'restricted definition requiring several symptoms or signs'. However, Lapkin and Golden (1978) also observed that basilar artery migraine was a common presentation in childhood. The variations partly reflect the different provenances of the various studies, and also the different interpretations placed upon the significance of 'difficult' symptoms such as unsteadiness, giddiness and complaints such as 'my eyes go funny'. Basilar artery migraine is discussed more fully in Chapter 3.

The nature of the migraine subject

In the absence of clear definition of the migraine attack and failure to identify it as a syndrome epidemiologically, there has been a wealth of literature which attempts to define, or characterize, the migraine subject – again, with few satisfactory conclusions.

Some disorders of childhood can be accepted as unusual forms (variants) of migraine, or as migraine attacks in which headache is absent (equivalents). These are discussed in Chapters 3 and 4. In addition, there are some otherwise unexplained disorders, uncommon but important, which may or may not be alternative expressions or precursors of migraine, and these are discussed in Chapter 6.

More difficulty lies with features which have been attributed to the subject with migraine as 'marking' him in some way. These include statements about intelligence, social class and personality characteristics and also about associations with phenomena such as travel sickness and sleep disturbance: to the extent that these features have been recommended as useful in the diagnosis of headache disorders and migraine.

Socio-economic status, intelligence and personality

The many repeated suggestions in the older literature that children with migraine are of higher *socioeconomic status* and *intelligence* have not been confirmed by controlled or community-based unselected study (Bille, 1962; Waters, 1971; Deubner, 1977; Goldstein and Chen, 1982; Kurtz *et al.*, 1984; Passchier and Orlebeke, 1985). Further, it appears unlikely that there are *personality* or *behavioural* traits which help define the migraine subject in any specific way. Bille (1962), and many others, have written about special personality characteristics of children with migraine, including features such as a greater tendency to anxiety, being 'more sensitive', more tidy, and more vulnerable to frustration, and showing less self-confidence than headache-free control groups. However, the recent study by Cunningham *et al.* (1987) stressed the need for control observations to include assessments made in children who were headache-free but who had experience of other longstanding pain disorders: they compared 20 migraine children with 20 children matched for age and sex, with chronic musculoskeletal pain, and 20 similarly matched children who were pain (and headache) free, but attending at the same hospital. When the amount of pain experienced by the children was controlled, the only discriminating variables between the groups were the specific somatic complaints, that is, there were no characteristics of the children with migraine other than their specific complaints of headache, nausea, etc. which could not have been accounted for by their experience of pain.

Sleep abnormality

Attempts to clarify the status of disordered sleep have not been successful, but this is not surprising where definitions of these disorders are not clear, nor likely to be single. For example, in a study of children attending a paediatric neurology clinic, Barabas *et al.* (1983a) found that 60 children with migraine headache (using Prensky's 1976 criteria) more often had *sleepwalking episodes* (30%) than 42 children with psychogenic, tension or post-traumatic headaches (4.8%), 60 children with seizure disorders (6.6%) and 60 with learning disability/perceptual or neurological impairment (5.0%). They suggested that disordered serotonin metabolism, being common to both disorders, could account for the increased frequency of sleepwalking in the migraine patients, and that its presence might be considered a criterion for migraine diagnosis. However, Bille (1962), in his large community study, did not find a higher incidence of somnambulism in his PMi group than in a control group of children, although when sleep disorders overall (night terrors, head banging and sleepwalking) were compared, these occurred more often in the PMi group. The subject is therefore still open and needs further study.

Motion sickness

It is similarly unclear whether migraine subjects are more prone to *motion sickness*. In the same groups of children referred to above, Barabas *et al.* (1983b) found that motion sickness (three or more episodes) occurred as an associated feature in 45% of their cases of childhood migraine, compared with only 5–7% of children with non-migraine headache, seizure disorders and learning disability/neurological or perceptual impairment. The authors again proposed a common underlying neurotransmitter disorder in migraine and motion sickness, or hypersensitivity of peripheral receptors (semicircular canals) to motion in subjects who have experienced (possibly basilar) migraine, or both mechanisms, to account for the association. They also recommended use of motion sickness as a minor diagnostic criterion for migraine. Others also report a high incidence of motion sickness in the past history of children with migraine. Thus Bille (1962) observed a history of motion sickness more often in his PMi group (55%) than in a control group of headache-free children (32%). Similarly in a school community study, Small and Waters (1974) observed that the proportion of children with a history of travel sickness increased according to whether they had no headache, non-migraine headache or headache with one, two or three of the usual characteristic features of migraine (unilateral headache, nausea, aura). However, in a study in another school the same investigators (Moss and Waters, 1974), using the same methodology, found that 62% of headache-free girls gave a history of travel sickness, compared with 31% of girls having headache without specific migraine features, and 61%, 60% or 64% of those having headache with one, two or all three of the usual specific migraine characteristics. Also, in a large schools community study, Deubner (1977) did not find any significant excess of travel sickness in children with migraine (headache with two or more of the classical symptoms) over children with non-migraine headache, or no headache: 38% of the migraine group, 31% of the non-migraine headache group and 32% of the no headache group said they had been travel sick. An association with migraine was not apparent in either the subjects', or their parents', replies.

Thus it would appear unwise, on published data, to unite the phenomena of migraine and motion sickness, in any common pathogenesis, or in the diagnosis of one with the other. However, motion is a well-known precipitant of migraine attacks in some subjects. Congdon and Forsythe (1979) observed this in 9% of their large series and Bille (1962) observed the same in 15% of his children with severe migraine. It is possible that these cases form a specific aetiological subtype of migraine. If this is so, then failure to separate this syndrome from other forms of migraine, with other aetiologies, could well account for the confusion and disagreement in the literature. Again, until the causes and triggers of migraine are understood, this difficulty will remain. On this uncertain background, use of motion sickness as a criterion for migraine diagnosis would seem unwise clinically.

Tourette's syndrome

It has also been suggested that Tourette's syndrome is linked with migraine: Barabas *et al.* (1984) observed migraine in 26.6% of 60 patients, aged 5–21 years, who presented (consecutively) with Tourette's syndrome. Again it is possible that these cases form a subtype of migraine. This needs further study.

Prognosis

The immediate prognosis for childhood migraine would appear to be good in at least half of the cases. Prensky and Sommer (1979) observed that irrespective of what treatment was given, many of their patients had a more than 50% reduction in headache frequency in the 6 months after consultation. They concluded: 'in general, treatment had little influence on the natural history of the disease'. Sills *et al.* (1982), Forsythe *et al.* (1984) and Gillies *et al.* (1986) made similar observations during placebo controlled studies of the effects of clonidine, propranolol and pizotifen. Noronha (1985) comparing timolol with placebo found 'progressive reduction of attack frequency in both treatment groups irrespective of treatment given', and Santucci *et al.* (1986) made the same observation when comparing placebo and L-5-hydroxytryptophan. Salfield *et al.* (1987) observed marked improvement in children taking a high fibre diet, whether or not vasoactive amines were excluded. were excluded.

In the long term also, childhood migraine is generally thought to have a good prognosis. However, this is not established, although it is recognized that long remissions occur. In a study of 102 migraine patients diagnosed before age 20, and reviewed after between 8 and 25 years (Hockaday, 1978), attacks had ceased in 29% of subjects having common migraine, 42% of those with basilar artery migraine, and 20% of those with visual, sensory or motor aura (26% of the series overall). Substantial improvement, in attack frequency or severity, or both, occurred in a further 48%. Only 17% were unchanged or worse, the remainder were unclear. Males outgrew their attacks more readily than females. However, sometimes there were long remissions followed by recurrence: 11% of patients still having attacks had experienced remissions exceeding 4 years, and 3% had experienced over 10 years' freedom before attacks recurred. One must question therefore whether migraine ever remits permanently. Congdon and Forsythe (1979) observed 65 (29%) of 228 children followed for more than 9 years had achieved an 8-year remission. Bille (1982) found 34% of children free from attacks 6 years after first ascertainment, and 41% free at 16 years of follow-up; by age 30 years or more, however, 60% of the series were still having attacks although many had been free for a period in their second or third decade. Sillanpää (1983a) reported that migraine starting before age 8 improved or ceased by age 14 in 58% of cases, although the later outcome in this epidemiological study is not yet known. Tal *et al.* (1984) reported that the majority (65%) of 73 children followed for a mean period of 5.4 years had become free from migraine (35) or had only mild infrequent headaches (12). Outcome is discussed further in Chapter 5.

Symptomatic migraine

A diagnosis of migraine implies the absence of demonstrable pathology. Sometimes, however, migraine, or a syndrome indistinguishable from it on clinical grounds, is symptomatic of underlying disease. *Symptomatic migraine* is rare, but important.

Vascular malformation

While it remains uncertain from published statistics whether the association between migraine and intracranial vascular malformations is greater than can be expected from chance (Lance, 1982), migraine-like syndromes undoubtedly occur in association with *vascular malformations*. The possibility that 'migraine' is symptomatic of an underlying vascular lesion should be considered if the headache is always confined to the same side, if the aura is stereotyped or prolonged, or shows a 'march', or if there are abnormal neurological signs or a cranial bruit, or if there are any seizures either with the headache or at other times. Although occasional patients diagnosed in later life as having a malformation have had headaches from early childhood, these are usually distinguishable. For example, the patient reported by Troost *et al.* (1979) had a stereotyped prolonged aura, and headache always on the same side, for 13 years prior to diagnosis at age 20 of an occipital arteriovenous malformation (all symptoms remitted after its removal).

Migraine symptomatic of an underlying vascular lesion is rare. In a large series of 500 patients with recurrent headache of vascular type, no example of a vascular malformation was found (Selby and Lance, 1960). Seventeen migraine patients had angiograms performed, because of persistent EEG focus (three), 'suspicious' plain X-ray (three), ophthalmic migraine (two), hemiparesis accompanying attacks (two), Jacksonian fits (one), solely for unilateral bruit (one), unilateral headaches (five): all were normal. In the series overall, an intracranial bruit was audible on auscultation over the orbits in ten cases – the bruit was unilateral in four, and three of these had normal angiograms. Lees (1962) reported that 23 of 300 consecutive unselected patients with migraine were considered to require angiography: this showed normal findings in all. In the same paper he analysed 50 cases of cerebral angioma, finding only 11 in whom recurrent headaches were the first symptoms. First symptoms/signs in the remainder were haemorrhage (42), epilepsy (nine), paresis (five), scotoma (one), aphasia (one), face pain (one). Three (possibly four) had symptoms which might have been interpreted as migraine, but were distinguishable because headache, and other focal symptoms, always affected the same side ('fixed migraine'). In the remaining eight cases, there were features excluding migraine (abnormal neurological signs, absence of any of the sensory phenomena of migraine, or early complications such as haemorrhage or epilepsy), and not one case completely simulated idiopathic migraine. Mackenzie (1953) had reached similar conclusions from a study of 50 patients with angioma. Twelve had headaches 'as long as they could remember': seven were 'migrainous', but none of these would have been diagnosed as migraine, because they showed atypical symptoms (consistent lateralization of headache/aura, prolonged aura, epilepsy) and four had a bruit. Others have reported rare examples where investigation of 'atypical' or complicated migraine has demonstrated an underlying vascular malformation. Pearce and Foster (1965) found two cases of angioma among 40 patients with complicated migraine: in both, attacks were marked by loss of consciousness, and one had seizures. Similarly, Slatter (1968) observed that five of 184 patients had grand mal epilepsy during their migraine: one was found to have an underlying angioma. Migraine-like headache is also reported in atypical Sturge–Weber syndrome (without visible naevus) (Battistella *et al.,* 1987).

Viral meningitis

Migraine may be symptomatic of *viral meningitis*. Rossi *et al.* (1985) discussed a 'benign migraine like syndrome with CSF pleocytosis', reviewing 23 cases reports, and describing four more cases in children of classic or hemiplegic migraine with elevated CSF cells, or protein, or both. They considered the possibility either that an underlying (viral) meningitis in some way triggered migraine attacks in susceptible subjects, or that the CSF abnormalities were secondary to the migraine; they favoured the latter explanation in most. They postulated a sterile inflammatory reaction to the release of excessive polypeptides in the CSF during migraine. However, Casteels-van Daele *et al.* (1981) had reported a child in whom CSF pleocytosis was observed on three separate occasions, in separate attacks of 'basilar migraine', with virus isolation from one specimen only: they concluded that the attacks in their case were indeed syptomatic of viral meningitis. Thus a viral aetiology should be sought very intensively.

Cerebral contusion

Syndromes clinically indistinguishable from migraine may occur following *cerebral contusion* (see Chapters 3 and 6). Sometimes the migraine may be accepted still as idiopathic, with the injury provoking an attack – as in footballer's migraine where heading the football is followed immediately by classical migraine (Matthews, 1972) – although this is not a very common phenomenon. However, there are reports of more severe neurological symptoms following relatively minor (non-concussive) head injury and occurring after a latent interval. Haas *et al.* (1975) described 50 such attacks in 25 subjects, 40 occurring in young subjects from 4 to 14 years, in which severe but transient neurological symptoms including hemiparesis, somnolence, irritability and vomiting, blindness or brainstem signs occurred after a latent interval of up to some hours. Some of the subjects had previously or at follow-up similar *spontaneous* attacks which were regarded as migraine. In another report Menken (1978) described transient confusion following minor head injury in two young subjects considered on other grounds to have migraine. It is of interest also that in two of four cases of acute confusional migraine described by Emery (1977), and in one of four described by Ehyai and Fenichel (1978) the neurological syndrome followed minor head injury. In these cases, the onset after a lucid latent interval suggests that local contusion might cause a local disruption of vasomotor control, with local tissue fluid changes, and initiation perhaps of spreading inhibition (of Leão) leading into migraine secondary to the focal brain injury. Alternative possibilities which would need to be considered and excluded before accepting such a 'migrainous' pathogenesis, include cerebral arterial or venous thrombosis (arterial thrombosis was demonstrated in two cases of four subjected to angiography by Haas *et al.* (1975)), and diffuse brain swelling, which may follow at an interval after trivial head injury in children (Bruce, 1984).

Metabolic disorders

There are a number of *metabolic encephalopathies* which present with recurrent or 'periodic' syndromes, often with nausea, vomiting, abdominal pain, confusion, and sometimes with headache. In most, it is unlikely that the disorder would be confused with migraine, provided that the essential criteria for diagnosis of migraine – its paroxysmal nature, with normal growth and development, and full return to normal health between attacks – are met. However, if the diagnosis of migraine is extended to undefined concepts such as abdominal migraine, then difficulty can follow (see Chapter 4). In particular, urea cycle disorders, aminoacidopathies, and mitochondrial cytopathies need to be considered in all otherwise unexplained recurrent syndromes of vomiting, whether or not there is associated lethargy or confusion. These topics are well reviewed by Adams and Lyon (1982) and Lloyd and Scriver (1985). Dvorkin *et al.* (1987) have written about a syndrome related to the mitochondrial encephalomyopathies, which they term 'malignant migraine', in which classical migraine is prominent, predating or coinciding with seizures and progressing cerebral disease. The difficulty this may cause in diagnosis, and the overlap between this syndrome and the syndrome of mitochondrial encephalopathy lactic acidosis, and stroke-like episodes (MELAS syndrome, Pavlakis *et al.*, 1984) is discussed further in Chapter 6.

Other forms of migraine

Many forms other than common and classical migraine are recognized in childhood. Some *special forms or variants,* for example basilar artery migraine, are relatively common, others such as ophthalmoplegic and hemiplegic forms are rare (Chapter 3). Migraine without headache is described in children, rarely as a recurrent neurological aura – *abortive migraine,* or migraine dissociée – and perhaps more commonly but much less specifically as recurrent extracranial visceral/vegetative symptoms – *migraine equivalents* (Chapter 4).

In addition, in infancy and early childhood a number of other paroxysmal disorders occur which have been described by some authors as precursors or *alternative expressions* of migraine, for example, the alternating hemiplegia syndrome, benign recurrent torticollis and benign paroxysmal vertigo (Chapter 6).

All these presentations carry very wide implications for differential diagnosis and are discussed in the relevant chapters.

Other causes of headache

Brief descriptions are given here of the major causes of headache in children. For a fuller review, and discussion of the differential diagnosis of headache syndromes in childhood, reference should be made to Barlow (1984).

Constitutional upset

Constitutional upset is probably the commonest cause of headache in children (Dalessio, 1987b). Headache can accompany fever of any cause. While it may be the only symptom complained of, it is usually just part of a recognizable clinical picture which is apparent on examination. Kandt and Levine (1987) noted that ill children attending a 'walk-in' paediatric clinic with complaints including headache were more likely to be febrile (30%) than were headache-free controls (11%), although diagnoses in the two groups were similar (e.g. pharyngitis, urinary tract infection). The children who experienced headache with their illness were also more likely to have a family history of migraine ($P \leqslant 0.05$), and the authors suggested that a tendency to fever-induced headache was an indication of possible future migraine.

Intracranial infection

Although drowsiness, irritability and photophobia can occur in any child with fever, and in the course of severe migraine, these symptoms also suggest intracranial infection: bacterial and viral meningitis, encephalitis, intracranial abscess. They are thus indications for special investigation especially in a child with headache, whether or not there is fever, or vomiting. Headache is a common early (prodromal) symptom in herpes simplex encephalitis. Symptoms of raised intracranial pressure (vomiting or alteration of conscious level), or evidence of focal neurological involvement, suggest intracranial abscess: failure to demonstrate any infection source does not rule this out; sometimes all that is found is sinusitis (Idriss *et al.*, 1978). In subacute and chronic meningitis, headache may be more insidious. Tuberculous meningitis is reported still in children in the UK (Naughten *et al.*, 1981), and in young children the history of headache, lethargy and anorexia may exceed 3 weeks (Fitzsimons, 1963).

Trauma

In younger children with head injury trauma may not be remembered, and this will be the case at any age when there is retrograde amnesia. Therefore, every child presenting with headache must be carefully examined for bruising. Non-accidental injury should be considered if the circumstances are unclear. Roberton *et al.* (1982) found head and facial bruising much more often in children in whom non-accidental injury was considered likely than in other traumatized children of the same age.

Occasionally minor trauma will cause haemorrhage from an underlying vascular malformation and this should be considered when headache of acute onset is prolonged, or increases in severity or when associated symptoms of neck stiffness, drowsiness or vomiting appear. Sometimes relatively minor trauma causes disruption of CSF dynamics, and leads to symptoms of headache, drowsiness and vomiting for the first time in children who have a previously balanced hydrocephalus either in relation to a space-occupying lesion, or with so-called arrested congenital hydrocephalus (Gordon, 1977). Demonstration of a large head size will be an important guide to the latter possibility.

Head injury (sometimes without obvious fracture) is a known cause predisposing to pneumococcal meningitis in children, perhaps by spread of infection across disrupted meninges: this possibility should be considered in a child whose headaches start, or increase, a few days after head trauma. Swartz and Dodge (1965) observed this in four of 14 children.

Late post-traumatic headache has not been much studied in children, but a recent paper by Lanzi *et al.* (1985) found it common. Of 217 children sustaining head injury between ages 3 and 17 years, 29% had later recurrent headaches. The incidence after mild head injury did not exceed that in a control group, and the authors concluded that 'cranial trauma does not assume a pathogenetic or predisposing role . . . if not accompanied by loss of consciousness'. They considered that headache manifesting after mild head injury might be migraine which would in any case have become manifest even without the head injury. They observed the late onset of migraine after severe head injury to be 20%, compared with 6% after average, and only 2% after mild injury. Whether or not head injury causes migraine to occur where it would not otherwise have done so is unclear. Head injury may be an important well-remembered event, and thus may emerge misleadingly as an antecedent. Pietrini *et al.* (1987) recorded past head injury in four of 12 children with acute confusional migraine, and Hockaday and Rose (1987) noted it in four of 29 children with migraine of different forms. This aspect needs further study.

Venous thrombosis

Cerebral venous and dural sinus thrombosis causes often dramatic presentations with headache, followed by other neurological symptoms and signs. The subject is reviewed comprehensively by Hilton-Jones (1988). *Cranial dural sinus thrombosis* commonly presents with headache which may soon be followed by other symptoms or signs of raised intracranial pressure such as nausea, vomiting, papilloedema, visual loss and cranial nerve palsies. It may be secondary to local infection, or to altered blood coagulability, but often no cause is found (Bousser *et al.*, 1985). It is likely that venous sinus thrombosis underlies many cases of so-called benign intracranial hypertension – *pseudotumour cerebri* (raised intracranial pressure without apparent structural cause). In this disorder the history may be of gradual onset and prolonged, with headaches recurring over some months before presentation. The condition is not rare in children (Grant, 1971; Rush, 1983). Headache is also the most prominent early symptom in cortical venous thrombosis, but here is usually quickly followed by other symptoms, in particular early seizures and other signs of cortical irritation or infarction, and raised intracranial pressure.

Intracranial haemorrhage

Spontaneous intracranial haemorrhage is rare in childhood. The Carlisle survey (Brewis *et al.*, 1966) did not identify any cases of SAH in a 5-year period in the 0–19-year age-group, and in a review of the literature found only eight (0.5%) of 1624 patients with SAH were under 10 years old. In one childhood series (Sedzimer and Robinson, 1973), the causes of haemorrhage were rupture of saccular aneurysm (27), vascular malformation (16), or unknown (24). Familial intracranial aneurysm presenting by rupture in childhood was recently reported, and both familial and non-familial intracranial aneurysm reviewed, by ter Berg *et al.* (1987). Typical presentation of intracranial haemorrhage is with headache of increasing severity that is unresponsive to analgesics, followed by deterioration of conscious level. Wong *et al.* (1983) also found SAH rare in children, but stressed that underlying brain tumour should be suspected in children who present with SAH: cerebral tumour was found in 26% of 15 children who presented with SAH over a 20-year period.

Cerebral tumour

Although cerebral tumour is rare (average annual incidence 5.2 per 100 000 population age 0–9 years in the Carlisle study, Brewis *et al.*, 1966), together with tumours of the spinal cord it is the second commonest cause of childhood malignancy, after leukaemia (Registrar-General's Annual Report' 1985). At all ages except infancy headache is the most important symptom of brain tumour, especially of those in the posterior fossa, where 45% of childhood brain tumours arise (Schulte, 1984). Geissinger and Bucy (1971) observed headache in 100% of children with cerebellar astrocytoma, usually antedating disturbance of gait by some months. Honig and Charney (1982) found 72 out of 105 children with brain tumour had associated headaches, *which preceded neurological and/or ocular signs in at least 83%*. The headaches were occipital in 28%, unilateral in 22% and diffuse in 50%. Skull X-ray was normal in 46% at the time of diagnosis. The headache of brain tumour results from local traction, and from the indirect distorting effects of the hydrocephalus which is generally present by the time of diagnosis: Honig and Charney (1982) recorded vomiting in 78% of children with brain tumour headache, and papilloedema was present in 63% at time of diagnosis. Geissinger and Bucy (1971) observed papilloedema at presentation in 88% of children with cerebellar astrocytoma. There may be no specific features about the headache of brain tumour. Paroxysmal attacks may occur over many months (Novak and Moshe, 1985), and the course can be intermittent with long remission. The intensity may be mild, and the quality throbbing (Rushton and Rooke, 1962). Thus distinction from the headache of migraine, or of muscle tension, cannot safely be made from the character of the headache alone. The circumstances in which it occurs are more helpful, and include any cause of altered intracranial pressure such as cough, sneezing, straining, exercise, recumbency and sleep – thus morning headache or headache which actually wakes a child can be ominous. Honig and Charney (1982) observed this feature in 67% of their series. However, in a review of the characteristics of brain tumour headaches (all ages), Rushton and Rooke (1962) found this feature in only 25% of cases overall.

In young children and infants, the headache of brain tumour at first presentation is likely to be accompanied by irritability, restlessness, crying, vomiting, dislike of having the head touched, a bulging fontanelle, head enlargement, and a cracked-pot note on skull percussion. Papilloedema is uncommon in early infancy (Farwell et al., 1978). In older children associated warning symptoms and signs may be unnoticed until vomiting supervenes. Early, and therefore important accompaniments of raised intracranial pressure from any cause in childhood are the psychic changes: cerebration is slowed, learning is interfered with, there may be change in personality, appearance of depression, increased fatiguability, lethargy, failure of attention, and apathy. *There may only be a slowing of intellectual development rather than regression.* In addition, slowing of growth, and other endocrine effects can occur, and bed-wetting should arouse suspicion of diabetes insipidus. Honig and Charney (1982) found that 60 of 72 children with headache due to brain tumour were diagnosed within 4 months of onset of their headaches (42 within 2 months), and they considered that 11 of the remaining 12 had symptoms or signs which could have led to earlier diagnosis: these included small stature, polydipsia, alteration in character and frequency of headache, behavioural changes, blurring of vision and diplopia, and incoordination. However, Flores et al. (1986) observed considerable delay in the diagnosis of brain tumour in children, particularly when contrasted with the early diagnosis made in tumour forms such as Wilms' tumour, and acute leukaemia. Again, headache was the commonest presenting symptom in 46 children age 6–20 years (61%). The mean interval from the appearance of symptoms to diagnosis was 26 weeks.

Children with headaches should therefore be observed long enough to establish that normal physical growth and intellectual and motor development continue, that performance of all skills is maintained, and that the child shows no alteration in personality or behaviour, over at least a 6-month period, with occasional review thereafter. Information obtained from school reports should be included in follow-up assessment.

Hydrocephalus

The more severe forms of hydrocephalus, and those associated with neural tube defect, present in infancy, but some of the congenital and posthaemorrhagic or postinfective types may not present until well into childhood; poor intellectual and motor performance generally predate headache in such children, but their significance may not be fully appreciated unless the large head size is noticed. In some cases, e.g. narrowing of the aqueduct of Sylvius (whether previously shunted or not), there may be periodic decompensation, and presentation with recurrent paroxysms of headache and vomiting. Others may have a more gradual build-up in pressure with low-grade chronic headache, not always obvious in very young children. It has been suggested (Smith, 1981) that children in whom the head size is large, either in absolute terms or relative to height, may have mild degrees of hydrocephalus manifesting only as cognitive problems; this has not been established (Gillberg and Rasmussen, 1982).

Ocular causes

Extraocular muscle imbalance with or without refractive error and overaccommo-dation can cause ocular discomfort, with headache in and around the eyes, and radiating to the frontal and temporal areas (Behrens, 1978). The frequency of headache attributable to these causes is probably overestimated, but ophthalmic examination should always be done. The commonest findings are uncorrected hyperopia, astigmatism and convergency insufficiency; glaucoma has been described.

Sinusitis

Acute sinusitis is usually self-evident, and accompanying local pain and tenderness reveal the site of infection. Headache with catarrh or chronic sinusitis, especially frontal, is more difficult to evaluate; many turn out to be of muscle tension type in children with allergic rhinitis (Birt, 1978). Finally nasopharyngeal malignancy, although very rare, can occur in children.

Cluster headache

Cluster headache is a severe form of unilateral head or facial pain which is typically associated with ipsilateral autonomic changes (lacrimation, nasal obstruction). The pain is usually fronto-orbital, and recurs once or more daily, typically at night, for a period of weeks or months, with a tendency for the pain to occur in bouts with long intervals of complete freedom. It should be considered as a separate entity from migraine (Lance, 1982). The condition rarely starts in childhood, but cases (usually male) as young as 6 years have been described (Del Bene and Poggioni, 1987; M. J. Noronha, 1987, personal communication).

Other causes

Other important conditions which may present in childhood as recurrent headaches include depressive illness (Ling *et al.*, 1970), arterial hypertension (Still and Cottom, 1967), phaeochromocytoma, psychomotor and other forms of epilepsy (see Chapter 7) and insulinoma. The relationships between hypoglycaemia and headache were discussed by Hockaday (1975). Temporomandibular joint dysfunction is reported as causing head and facial pain in children, with a strong association with depression (Belfer and Kaban, 1982). Headache can also occur as a true conversion (hysterical) symptom. This is a clinically important diagnosis needing urgent psychiatric management; the selective nature of the limitation of activity and the disability is usually striking. Psychogenic or assumed headache is another common 'headache' presentation. School refusal is an important underlying cause of these syndromes.

Headache due to cervical and scalp muscle tension resulting from anxiety is rare in very young children but can occur in middle childhood years, and is common in older children and juveniles. Distinction from common migraine may be impossible, and often both coexist. Children with headache of tension type are often pale, and they may be anorexic; they rarely complain of nausea or vomiting.

Conclusion

When there are abnormal physical signs, or neurological symptoms, then the nature of these will guide investigation. When headache is unaccompanied by other symptoms, and ordinary clinical examination does not show any abnormality, then the problem is of *unexplained headache*. While most unexplained headache in childhood is migraine, or tension or psychogenic headache, there must always be concern at first presentation that a structural lesion may underlie the symptoms. In general, unexplained headache should be investigated further if headache attacks become more severe, more prolonged or more frequent, if the pain is not relieved by mild painkilling drugs, if there is any suggestion that the child's personality or behaviour is altering, or that normal developmental milestones are becoming retarded, if physical growth is not maintained, and if the head circumference exceeds the normal centile lines, or is considerably out of line with height. The appearance of visual or neurological symptoms, or of abnormal signs on examination of course will also indicate need for special investigation. These guidelines imply the need for continuing observation for a period, to establish continued well-being, growth, and development.

Summary

Migraine of common or classical form occurs in 3–5% of boys and girls, from an early age. Before puberty boys slightly outnumber girls. Headache attacks last typically a few hours, but may be brief, of half an hour's duration or less, and occasionally continue over 24 h. Many other forms of migraine occur: special forms or variants of migraine, abortive migraine and equivalents of migraine, and, in addition, some paroxysmal disorders of early childhood which it is suggested may be alternative forms, or precursors, of migraine.

Diagnosis of migraine can be difficult. Definition by criterion is not satisfactory for clinical use in childhood, and diagnosis is by exclusion of other causes of recurrent headache. It depends more on the circumstances, and the temporal pattern, of attacks than on the actual characteristics of the headache itself, and requires a period of observation during which it can be established that the child remains otherwise well, and that growth and development continue normally.

Disability from common and classical migraine is not often severe, frequent school absence is rare, and prognosis for at least temporary regression of attacks is good. However, in infants and children, as in adults, occasional severe forms occur, with considerable disability, and, sometimes, morbidity.

Chapter 2

Epidemiology and inheritance of migraine in children

Dewey K. Ziegler

Prevalence

Only within recent decades have epidemiological studies confirmed the fact that headache is an extremely frequent symptom in children. Studies have been done in Scandinavia and the UK. The classic one is that of Bille (1962) who carefully surveyed by questionnaire, and often by interview, a community sample of 8993 Swedish children. In this population only 3720 said they had never had headache, another 4316 said they had had headache seldom (never 'paroxysmal'). Three studies have been carried out in Finland. In the study of Sillanpää (1976) of 4235 7-year-old children before starting school, 37.7% had experienced headache with 13.3% reporting headache at a frequency of greater than once a month. A later study (Sillanpää, 1983b) of 3784 schoolchildren aged 13 found that 87% had suffered headache in the previous year, headache being defined as 'pain in the area of the head which handicapped the pupil's school attendance, homework, free-time activities of daily living'. Another study in Finland (Sillanpää and Piekkala, 1984) of 3863 14-year-olds found 94.2% of this population recorded headache, which in 32% was 'disturbing' and recurred at least monthly in the previous year. Small and Waters (1974) found in a British community sample aged 10–16 years severe headaches reported at least once a month by 27.3% of girls and 27.2% of boys. Another British study (Collin *et al.*, 1985) recording school records over two school terms of children aged 5–14 years found 3.6% had missed school because of headache during this period. Oster (1972) in a similar large school population, aged 6–19 years, found the prevalence overall of 'suffering from headache' was 20.6%. In summary it can be said that headache is not rare in children and prevalence probably increases with increasing age (see Table 1.1).

There is little information from other societies and other cultures – data which would be of great interest because of the reported discrepancy in prevalence of headache in adults of different cultures (Ogunyemi, 1984; Sachs *et al.*, 1985; Cheng *et al.*, 1986). As noted, the large population studies on children have been done chiefly in Scandinavia and Britain where there are fairly homogeneous ethnic populations. Studies citing frequencies in black and white children have been from comparatively small selected populations (e.g. Rigg, 1975). Whether prevalence of childhood headache varies with socioeconomic class has only been studied infrequently. Bille (1962) did not find difference in migraine frequency in different social classes. The National Child Development Study in Great Britain (Kurtz *et al.*, 1984) investigating, in a large cohort of children, a wide variety of illnesses including migrainous and non-migrainous 'sick headache' found that 'those with non-migrainous headache were more likely to come from disadvantaged home backgrounds'. Significant associations were found with a father in manual occupation and an environment showing signs of poverty.

There is also little data on the change in overall headache prevalence at different childhood ages, although some follow-up data to be discussed later bears on this point. Bille (1962) reported gradually increasing prevalence throughout the first decade. Sillanpää and Piekkala (1984), studying the same population group of children at age 13 and 14, found a rise in headache prevalence and speculated that the increase could be due to the stress of moving to a higher school level.

Problems of definition

By far the largest part of the epidemiological literature on this subject concerns itself not with undefined headache but with headache of migrainous type. Since there are no objective tests by which headache disease entities may be identified, it has proven difficult to obtain a consensus on the definition of migraine. It has been known since antiquity that the pain of severe headache is commonly unilateral, and commonly associated with nausea and vomiting. However, it is only within the past few decades that attention has been focused on how commonly these variables are associated, and how commonly they are associated with the visual phenomena that define classical migraine (Lance and Anthony, 1966; Waters, 1973). There have been at least three commonly used definitions, that of Vahlquist (1955), that of the Ad Hoc Committee of the American Academy of Neurology (1962), and that of the World Federation of Neurology (1969). There have also been several others, e.g. that of Prensky and Sommer (1979). Although the definitions are in general similar, they differ somewhat in the variables included; all include language which demands subjective judgement, e.g. the terms 'commonly' and 'frequently'. Clinical aspects of definition are discussed in Chapter 1.

Problems in definition may account for some of the variation in findings of migraine prevalence in children. Figures from 2% to 10% have been reported. Bille (1962) found in his population of 8993 children, 'paroxysmal' headaches in 484. The definition problem is clearly illustrated by the fact that attacks in 103 of these children included one additional migraine characteristic, 160 included two, 130 included three, and 57 all four. The interesting observation relevant to definition was made that, if three criteria were considered essential to the diagnosis, 60 cases with visual aura (certainly the most specific of the migraine characteristics) would have been ruled out. Dalsgaard-Nielsen et al. (1970) in a community survey of migraine in 2027 schoolchildren and adolescents 7–19 years of age found a mean migraine prevalence of 2.9% in the 7–9 year age-group, with the figure gradually and steadily rising throughout childhood. The Finnish study (Sillanpää, 1976) found 3.2% of a population of 7-year-olds having recurrent headache with two or more features of migraine. In the large study by Oster (1972) of children aged 6–19 years, incidence of migraine (exact defining criteria not given) was 4.6% in boys and 6.4% in girls. A British survey of schoolchildren aged 10–18 reported migraine in 3.3% of boys and 2.5% of girls (Sparks, 1978). However, these figures are suspect because they derive from a voluntary answer to a questionnaire and there is no information on those who did not reply. An additional problem, rarely mentioned, is that in the same individual the percentage of headache attacks with one or more of the above characteristics may vary widely; e.g. a small percentage may be accompanied by a visual aura. Finally, this percentage is characteristically not constant over time; e.g. the percentage of attacks with nausea and vomiting may be high one year and low the next.

Childhood features

Several studies have documented that migraine can, uncommonly, have its onset in the first few years of life (Vahlquist and Hackzell, 1949; Burke and Peters, 1956; Bille, 1962). Children, who later have typical attacks, have been noted in the preverbal stage to have attacks characterized by nausea and signs of autonomic dysfunction and gestures indicating head pain. In an adult series, Selby and Lance (1960) found 21% reported onset before 10 years, and 25% between 10 and 20 years. In a childhood series, Hockaday (1979) found onset by age 7 years in 62% and by age 10 years in 86%, and Congdon and Forsythe (1979) observed onset before age 5 years in one-third of their children.

The mean age of onset of migraine in boys is earlier than that in girls (Bille, 1962; Dalsgaard-Nielsen et al., 1970), but remissions in childhood occur as will be noted later. Childhood migraine differs from adolescent and adult migraine in several ways. Possibly the most interesting is sex difference. Whereas in adults migraine predominates in women by a factor of at least 2 to 1 (far more in several series), in childhood this is not true. In early childhood there is either a slightly increased percentage of boys (Bille, 1962; Dalsgaard-Nielsen et al., 1970; Sillanpåå, 1976) or an equal sex frequency (Oster, 1972). The female preponderance begins about age 12. It appears that this preponderance may correlate with menarche (Epstein et al., 1975).

In two British studies Waters and his colleagues investigated the prevalence of headache and of each of three major features of migraine in two large school groups aged 10–16 years. Some headache in the previous year was reported in 85–90%, with 36% of girls and 29% of boys reporting severe headache. Very high percentages reported one or more of the migrainous features, e.g. 82–87% of the girls reported unilateral distribution, over half of both sexes reported nausea (Moss and Waters, 1974; Small and Waters, 1974). Waters (1974b) discussed the problems of reliability for different symptoms and for data from different sources.

Nausea, vomiting and other abdominal symptoms are a more universal part of childhood migraine attacks than of those of adults. Some have stated that unilateral head pain is less prominent in children, but others have questioned whether this finding may not have been artefactual in that children may not be as accurate in this detail as adults.

There is also disagreement as to whether the visual scotomata defining classical migraine are more or less common in children. At least three series of migrainous children (clinic samples) state that visual aura is uncommon and reviews have stated the same fact (Burke and Peters, 1956; Rigg, 1975; Prensky and Sommer, 1979). The community study of Bille however reports it occurring in approximately 25% of children with 'paroxysmal' headache and that of Sillanpåå (1976, 1983b) in 21% of his 7-year-old population and in 74% of the 'paroxysmal' headache group of his 13-year-old population.

Because of case rarity it is uncertain how specifically migraine associated with confusional states or states of altered awareness is particularly characteristic of childhood, although most cases seem to have had onset in early life. Such states include a variety of abnormalities of consciousness, cognitive function and perception. There is, for example, the distortion of visual perception that has been called the 'Alice in Wonderland' syndrome in which the child's perceptions are described in terms of Alice's perception of herself after eating the enchanted substance (Golden, 1979). Lewis Carroll, it is speculated, may have been speaking from personal experience. These forms of migraine are discussed in Chapters 3 and 7.

Other variants of migraine with features of neurological deficit other than seizures are rare, but may occur more commonly in childhood than in adult life, e.g. acute confusional states and transient global amnesia. Migraine associated with hemiplegia or ophthalmoplegia are variants that have long been observed but their exact frequency has not been documented. Ophthalmoplegic migraine is considered commonest in young children. A specific syndrome of alternating hemiplegia beginning in infancy with each attack occurring with contralateral headache has been described. There is little epidemiological data concerning these migraine variants, except the fact that, as noted, case reports suggest that their onset and frequency are more common in childhood and adolescence than in adult life (Rossi et al., 1980). They are fully discussed in Chapter 3.

Course

The course of childhood migraine has been seldom studied. Studies done, however, show that remissions are common. Bille (1962) found that after a 6-year follow-up period 51% of the children originally diagnosed as having migraine were free of this diagnosis and 31% had improved. Roughly the same percentage of improvement had occurred in a subgroup of the 73 whom he had designated 'pronounced migraine'. At later follow-up, after a further 10 years, 41% of these individuals were free of migraine, 32% improved, and 27% unimproved or worse (Bille, 1973). Of the original population with non-migrainous headache 69% were headache free, 19% improved and 12% had developed migraine. Hockaday (1978) reported cessation of migraine in 35% of male and 21% of female migraineurs after an interval of 8–25 years. Age of onset did not correlate with migraine cessation and many patients with continuing attacks reported prolonged clear intervals (e.g. 4–10 years). The EEG also did not correlate with outcome. Congdon and Forsythe (1979) in a follow-up of 300 children aged 5–14 years found that 29% had an 8-year remission and 34% a 10-year remission. None of these latter children had relapsed but a few did so after a 2- to 3-year remission. In a Mayo clinic study 9–14 years after treatment, 32.8% were completely free of headache and 46.6% considerably improved (Hinrichs and Keith, 1965).

In summary, there is a strong tendency for childhood migraine to remit, at least for several years. How frequently it recurs in adult life is documented apparently only in the two studies of Bille (1973) and Hockaday (1978). Bille (1981) reported that of his original 73 'pronounced migraine' group after 23 years, 60% were still having migraine attacks, a large number having been free for several years. It is also possible that a percentage of subjects with childhood classic migraine develop common migraine later in life, and vice versa as discussed above.

Whether the prevalence of migraine is linked to socioeconomic status has rarely been studied. In adults, Waters (1971) could find no difference. The National Child

Development study in Britain found, as noted previously, that children with 'sick headaches' were more likely to come from poor home backgrounds (Kurtz *et al.*, 1984): however, only 27% of this group were considered to have migraine, and data on this subgroup is not presented separately.

Associations

Paroxysmal vertigo

The possible association of childhood migraine with other non-painful episodic symptoms has been the subject of much study. One of the most common of these is paroxysmal vertigo. Continental authors have written extensively about the association of vertigo and headache, and in recent years interest has focused on two aspects of this subject – the possible abnormality of the vestibular apparatus in these patients, and the relation to the specific entity of basilar artery migraine. There is a frequent clinical coincidence of paroxysmal vertigo and migraine, probably with specific increased frequency in children; it is rarely due to any demonstrable abnormality of vestibular function. This subject is discussed in full in Chapter 6.

Episodic abdominal pain

Even more complex is the relationship of episodic abdominal pain to headache. Recurrent abdominal pain is common in children, having been reported in from 10 to 18% of various population samples (Miller *et al.*, 1974; Small and Waters, 1974). It is said to be a frequent association with childhood migraine but this has not been established by epidemiological study. This subject is discussed in Chapter 4.

Allergy

One of the most interesting suggested associations is that of migraine with allergic diseases. A voluminous literature over past decades has asserted that 'migraine is an allergic disease' (Unger and Unger, 1952), but there have been few unselected population studies of the subject. In the British National Childhood Development Study (Kurtz *et al.*, 1984) an association was found between all children with headache and those with a current and past history of asthma. When a series of children with a variety of respiratory problems was studied, it was found that histories of migraine and recurrent abdominal pain were associated to a significant degree with wheezy bronchitis but not with asthma (Peckham and Butler, 1978).

Three studies in children, however, have suggested that there is a close connection between migraine and food allergy. In one study (Monro *et al.*, 1980) 25% of migrainous children were said to display food sensitivity. In another study by the same group, Bentley *et al.* (1984) reported that of 12 migrainous children with recurrent abdominal pain and a family history of classic migraine, four had eczema, and all were said to improve on an exclusion diet. In the third large study (Egger *et al.*, 1983) of 88 children with severe frequent migraine, 93% were found to recover on a diet excluding substances to which they had been found sensitive. Sequential reintroduction of suspected substances was said to provoke attacks. This last trial which was controlled and double blind, is persuasive and deserves replication. What the exact nature of the suggested association might be remains unknown. There is certainly rarely evidence of brain oedema in migraine attacks. The evidence concerning an immunological abnormality of serum complement in migraine remains controversial (Lord and Duckworth, 1978; Moore *et al.*, 1980). As in so many areas in migraine, an abnormality, even if present, may not relate to headache as a cause. It may be a parallel phenomenon deriving from an unknown common source. The subject is discussed more fully in Chapter 8.

Psychological variables

The relationship of migraine to psychological variables is an even more complex and contentious subject. In general, children with a variety of recurrent headaches have not been found to differ from controls in intelligence but there are reported characteristic personality qualities. In Bille's study (1962), for example, migrainous children were described by parents as more anxious, sensitive and more vulnerable to frustration than the control group children, and also more tidy and less physically enduring. Bille also found that migrainous children, particularly girls, approached tests with attitudes of restraint and cautiousness. Migrainous children, again more commonly girls, rated themselves, to a highly significant degree, as more subject to anxiety. In the National Child Development Survey (Kurtz *et al.*, 1984) one of the most striking findings was the high proportion of children with sick headaches who, in the 7-, 11- and 16-year age-groups, showed signs of emotional disturbance. 'Maladjustment or deviant behaviour' particularly at home was present to a highly significant degree. These findings parallel those of numerous investigators. Vahlquist (1955), for example, describes his findings in the following phrases: 'children with migraine more regularly than adults exhibit that special constitutional type which is characterized by neurovegetative instability, overdue ambition and perfectionism'. Krupp and Friedman (1953) in their 75 migrainous children noted the personality traits of ' . . . sensitivity, cleanliness, thoroughness, the need for approval and the need to take seriously such responsibilities as school and dress'. In another study (Stone and Barbero, 1970) children with recurrent abdominal pain and headache were described as 'sensitive . . . older than their years . . . dependent . . . constant worriers'. One controlled study of migrainous children (Maratos and Wilkinson, 1982) found a significantly higher proportion with a neurotic disorder (mainly anxiety or depression). This increased prevalence was found to be associated with a disturbed parental relationship.

Two other recent studies of children with 'idiopathic headache' compared to age-matched controls found 'feelings of being excluded from the family group, insecurity, and repressed hostility toward important figures' to be significantly stronger in the patients (Guidetti *et al.*, 1983), and a condition of 'repressed anger' preceding the attack in 85% of the cases (Lanzi *et al.*, 1983).

Depression has specifically been reported in migrainous children, with marked improvement by the use of amitriptyline (Ling *et al.*, 1970). However, doubts have been raised. A recent study (Cunningham *et al.*, 1987) measured anxiety and depression using four instruments: psychological scales, parent and teacher report forms, and pain diaries kept by children. Results were compared to two control groups – one with chronic musculoskeletal pain and a no-pain group. Results were similar in the migraine and pain group suggesting that the personality qualities alleged to be specific for migraine are in fact the result of chronic pain. However, the study does not completely invalidate previous findings of personality traits common in migraine.

Naturally it is of interest that the qualities described are similar to those cited in the past for adult migraineurs by, for example, Wolff (Dalessio, 1987a) and Alvarez (1947), and there is currently similar uncertainty about the existence in adults of a significant association with migraine. If these personality qualities are peculiar to migraine, the connection to headache remains totally unknown. Numbers of interesting unsolved questions are raised by these psychological studies. Do these personality qualities correlate in any way with migraine types, or with EEG patterns? Are variables in personality patterns associated in any significant way with variations in the life-history of migraine? What is the relationship, if any, between personality qualities and the provocation of a headache attack by a certain stimulus, be it 'emotional stress', or some other factor, biochemical, physiological or environmental?

Inheritance

In most studies of migraine, increased prevalence of headache in family members has been recorded – to such a degree that a family history has often been used as a diagnostic criterion. It appears that such 'positive family histories' are more common in migraine having onset in childhood (Bille, 1962). One controlled study, however, has disputed the fact of increased prevalence of headache in relatives of migraineurs (Waters, 1971).

The exact nature of a genetic factor has long been disputed. In the past dominant, recessive and sex-linked patterns of inheritance have been postulated, although in many typical cases, there is no evidence of a genetic element. Barolin and Sperlich (1969) favoured a polygenetic mechanism and a recent study using segregation analysis also came to the conclusion that the data did not support the hypothesis of a single gene (Devoto et al., 1986).

Several studies have been done in twins to determine if there is increased concordance of migraine in monozygotic twin pairs. Results illustrate the complexity of the problem. A Danish questionnaire study (Harvald and Hauge, 1956) of 1900 twin pairs found concordance for migraine in six of 12 monozygotic twin pairs but in only three of 27 dizygotic twin pairs, and the comment was made that, due to the methodology of the study, 'the figures for concordance must therefore also be regarded as minimum figures'. Two other smaller studies, however, did not find increased concordance in monozygotic twins (Schepank, 1974; Ziegler et al., 1975). To avoid the problem of migraine definition, the study of Ziegler et al. (1975) looked for concordance in pairs where one individual gave a history of any severe or incapacitating headache. Zygocity in this study was verified by blood typing. Again, in this study increased concordance was not found in monozygotic twin pairs compared to dizygotic same-sex controls (Ziegler et al., 1975). The most recent large twin study of Lucas (1977) found a concordance rate of 26% in monozygotic twins and 13% in controls, a significant difference ($P < 0.05$). Zygocity was determined clinically however, and the author found in a small sample with blood group checking that 6% clinically determined as monozygotic were indeed dizygotic. The Lucas study (1977) also investigated possible concordance for specific clinical features and found significantly more concordance in monozygotic twins for neurological prodromata (e.g. scintillating scotomata), 'steady headache' and 'sickness' (nausea). However, the author comments that neither headache in general nor any specific symptom showed a very high concordance. Others have reported monozygotic twin pairs with striking concordance of migraine symptomatology (Juel-Nielsen, 1965).

To summarize, twin data substantiate the hypothesis that there is some genetic element in migraine but that it is less important than generally thought.

There have been no systematic studies comparing small groups of migrainous children with and without affected relatives and with the emphasis on certain well-defined variables to determine if there might be a more clear genetic pattern in such groups. The composition of a genetic factor predisposing to migraine is totally unknown. There is evidence in various populations of inheritance of personality traits (Loehlin, 1982), visual, auditory and somatosensory evoked responses (Lewis *et al.*, 1972), and various enzymes, e.g. monoamine oxidase (Pandey *et al.*, 1979), a few of the factors that may contribute to the predisposition to headache. These and many other genetic traits may interact with each other or with environmental variables to produce various clinical headache syndromes, e.g. migraine.

Migraine and other neurological disorders

Epilepsy

The possible relationship of migraine and epilepsy continues a vexed subject since Gowers made the famous connection in his monumental text (Gowers, 1907). It has recently been considered at length by Andermann and Lugaresi (1987).

A genetic relationship between migraine and epilepsy has long been asserted, and Lennox and Lennox (1960) reported increased prevalence of seizures in relatives of migrainous patients. However, a genetic relationship has been denied by other reports. In one recent study (Baier, 1985) of 81 patients with childhood onset of migraine, interviews with siblings, parents and grandparents were carried out. No increase in seizures over that in a control group was found in any type of migraine. However, in another report from the same institution (Baier and Doose, 1987), the surprising finding is reported that in maternal relatives, and in particular mothers of *female* children with absence seizures, there is a high prevalence of migraine – significantly higher than in maternal relatives of male patients. There is again the possibility of bias in case selection, although it is difficult to see why migrainous mothers of girls, as opposed to boys, would be seen in the clinic. In the very useful study of Kraus (1978), quoted in detail by Andermann and Andermann (1987), prevalences of migraine in relatives of epileptic and control probands were the same.

Thus at the present time there is no consistent evidence of a genetic link between migraine and epilepsy. However, there are a number of other ways in which migraine and seizures of different sorts may be linked, and a number of conditions in which the distinction between migraine and epilepsy may be difficult. (For further discussion see Chapter 7.)

Somnambulism

In children with migrainous headache Giroud *et al.* (1986) reported a highly significant percentage with a history of somnambulism but no such correlation with non-migrainous headache. These findings would correlate with the occurrence of sleep-precipitated headache, in Stages III and IV, and in rapid eye movement (REM) sleep (Dexter and Weitzman, 1970).

Learning disorders

Leviton (1986) has recently reported that sizable percentages of children with migraine have had academic difficulty prior to the onset or with exacerbation of headache. As noted above, there have been many studies of emotional states of children with migraine, but few with fine tuned evaluation of cognitive function. This observation awaits confirmation.

Other headache

Apart from the problem of migraine is the broader question of headache in general. Certainly far more frequent than classic migraine and probably more frequent than common migraine is the group of headache symptoms formerly called tension headache and currently 'muscle contraction'. A recent review (Pikoff, 1984) has focused on the weakness of the evidence that these frequent longlasting painful symptoms are consistently associated with muscle tension. It has also been emphasized recently that typical migraine often evolves, in later years, into 'chronic daily headache'. The frequency of these events in children has not been studied. We have only overall figures on 'non-migrainous' headache. Whether these headaches are a part of a syndrome of a general tendency to headaches of which migraine is one variant, or whether they are indeed a syndrome apart, closely related to psychological disturbance, remains one of the central problems in paediatric as in adult migraine.

Conclusion

The epidemiology of childhood migraine suggests several problems of particular interest:

1. Is the change from an equal sex ratio to one of marked female preponderance in the second decade related to menarche in women?
2. Does the childhood pattern of migraine (e.g. the percentage of classic attacks) persist into adult life?
3. What is the significance of the increased percentage of childhood migraine with EEG abnormalities?
4. Is the migraine–allergy connection more firm in childhood than adult life?
5. Is the epidemiology of childhood migraine more or less uniform worldwide?

At present answers to these questions are, at the least, indefinite. Further research needs to define more homogeneous populations of children with headache. A consistent correlation of a clinical headache syndrome with some measurable biological or biochemical variable remains non-existent.

Summary

Headache is extremely common in childhood, and migraine, more narrowly defined, is also frequent, affecting probably 3–5% of the population. Unlike the situation in adults, migraine in childhood affects boys and girls with equal frequency. Migraine often has an extremely early onset and occasionally is associated with dramatic neurological dysfunction, e.g. confusion. Remissions are common. Episodic vertigo and abdominal pain occur in migrainous children. There are strong suggestions that allergies, particularly food allergies, play a role in some childhood migraine. There is some evidence that migrainous children are characterized by more psychological disturbances than controls, and may possess the obsessive-compulsive personality traits often attributed to adult migraineurs.

Although a history of affected relatives is common in migrainous children, the exact genetic role remains ill defined. There is no consistent evidence of a genetic link between migraine and epilepsy.

The relationship of migraine to muscle contraction headache in children, as in adults, remains controversial. Whether these syndromes are indeed separate entities or variations on a common theme is still an unsolved problem.

Chapter 3

Special forms: variants of migraine in childhood

Gwilym Hosking

Introduction

A special form or *variant* of migraine is one which is unusual because of the nature of the neurological symptoms and signs associated with the attack, but which otherwise fulfills ordinarily acceptable criteria for diagnosis. The term is not nosologically exact, but is used here in preference to labels such as complicated migraine, or migraine accompagnée, often used in different ways by different authors. By definition, common migraine, and classical migraine with brief visual aura are excluded. Again by definition, equivalents of migraine (migraine without headache) are not under discussion here (see Chapter 4).

Unusual forms of migraine, with prominent or persisting specific neurological symptoms and signs, raise important questions for the clinician about differential diagnosis, and the need for special (often invasive) investigation.

The special forms of migraine that will be discussed here are those which have in the past been grouped together as 'complicated migraine', or 'migraine accompagnée or associée', terms originally employed by Piorry (quoted by Bruyn, 1986). Charcot reserved the term 'complicated migraine' for those instances in which the headache was accompanied by neurological deficits that were permanent (Bruyn, 1986). Neurological deficits that were recognized included dysphasia, hemianopia, scintillating scotoma, numbness, paresis, paraesthesiae, and cranial nerve palsy. While permanent deficits are well known, they are uncommon, and for the most part the associated neurological symptoms and signs – albeit unusual, profound, or prolonged – are transient, and this is recognized in current definitions. Thus Dalessio (1987a) uses the term 'complicated migraine' for cases in which focal neurological signs persist for 24 h or more beyond the headache phase but then subside, and Saper (1983) includes as complicated migraine attacks in which signs that occur during the headache phase persist through the attack, but then subside completely at the same time as the headache.

The more important and *specific* of these syndromes are discussed below. Certain special aspects, for example symptomatic migraine, and syndromes of altered mental state are also discussed in other chapters (see index). It is important to note however that although terminology and classification of special migraine syndromes imply that they are distinct, there is considerable variation in, and some overlap between, the presentations, and in most cases simpler forms of migraine also occur. Indeed, their occurrence, in association, or later, is essential in diagnosis.

Hemiplegic migraine and other hemisyndromes

While the earliest discussions about hemiplegic migraine centred on whether such a form of migraine existed, in the last few decades the debate has turned to the question of how many variants of hemiplegic migraine exist. Whatever that argument may be there seems to be at least a general acceptance that hemiplegic migraine can be defined as 'a vascular headache featured by sensory and motor phenomena which persist during and after the headache'.

The link with a positive family history of migraine has not been in dispute. However, in some reports it has been recognized that there may be a positive family history of common or classical migraine while in others it is of hemiplegic migraine. We thus have a measure of agreement in the existence of familial hemiplegic migraine, in which the history within the family is that of hemiplegic attacks alone, and of sporadic hemiplegic migraine in which other forms of migraine have occurred in family members. In the study by Bradshaw and Parsons (1965) the authors extended the scope of the term hemiplegic migraine to cover migrainous headaches associated with transient motor *or* sensory symptoms referred to one side. From this the authors suggested that hemiplegic attacks represented approximately 30% of migraine attacks as a whole, while Heyck (1969) with a more restrictive definition suggested 4% and Whitty (1986) 9%. Whatever figures are accepted none can be used to indicate what the population prevalence is of this form of migraine due to the inevitable problems of selection as well as of the clinical criteria accepted for the diagnosis (Whitty, 1986).

In common with a number of the other forms of migraine inheritance is more commonly from the maternal family, although possibly there is a higher paternal inheritance in females who display focal symptomatology. The frequency of positive family histories will vary, again due not only to the differing criteria accepted for the designation of hemiplegic migraine, but because of the inevitable selection of published reports (Bradshaw and Parsons, 1965). The incidence of positive family histories appears to range from about 18% to 60%. Overall there would appear *not* to be an increased incidence of positive family histories with complicated migraine as distinct from classical or common migraine.

Clinical presentations

While some have argued that the presentation of familial hemiplegia is at an earlier age, the episodes more stereotyped, prolonged and severe than in sporadic forms (Fenichel, 1985), others have suggested that there is no difference in either the presentation or clinical course between the two forms of attacks (Bradshaw and Parsons, 1965; Whitty, 1986). The age of onset of hemiplegic migraine is most usually in childhood and earlier than for common migraine. In a report of a family where ten members were affected, onset of attacks was in childhood in nine (Glista *et al.*, 1975). In many subjects hemiplegic attacks cease in adulthood, being replaced by other forms of attack (Jensen *et al.*, 1981a). In some patients an attack may be precipitated by minor trauma as may occur in association with football (heading the ball) or rugby football (a blow on the head or face as in a tackle). In some attacks may only occur in such situations although in most they occur at other times as well. Four groups of attacks have been described in association with minor trauma: (1) hemiparetic, (2) somnolence, irritability and vomiting, (3) transient blindness and (4) brainstem signs. The hemiparetic attacks seem to be frequently repeated and the onset of attacks is most usually 1–10 min after the trauma (Haas *et al.*, 1975; Ashworth, 1985).

The unilateral neurological signs and symptoms that characterize hemiplegic migraine most typically occur as part of the prodrome or as a manifestation of the migrainous aura. In many, but not all, they are confined to this phase of the attack. In these individuals the unilateral symptoms will be replaced by a contralateral hemicranial headache, or, in some, by bilateral, diffuse or even ipsilateral headache. In other patients, however, it may be the severe headache that commences first, combined perhaps with alteration in consciousness, to be followed shortly thereafter by steady progression of a hemisyndrome.

The frequency of visual symptoms in patients with hemiplegic migraine indicates that in a number there is involvement not only of the carotid territory but also of the posterior cerebral hemisphere. Indeed, it is relatively common for the attack to begin with visual symptoms in the ipsilateral field of vision (Heyck, 1973). These visual symptoms will vary in nature and may consist of either scintillating or simple scotomata.

Shortly after or at the same time as the onset of visual symptoms, usually over a period of minutes, there is an onset of unilateral sensory or motor symptoms involving initially the face and then the arm and to a lesser extent the leg. Paraesthesiae may occur with onset in the fingers or thumb, spreading into the hand and perhaps the forearm, and then involving the ipsilateral mouth, lips, tongue, or face (cheiro-oral migraine). For many the most dramatic symptom may be numbness but a slow progression of weakness is also characteristic. The rate of progression is slow when comparisons are made with the more rapid march of a seizure. Dysarthria is common in association with the hemiparesis, and – together with this – aphasia is also common in the early stages, seemingly irrespective of which side is affected.

Some alteration in consciousness is common in most attacks. This may range from mild confusion to coma and in some to frank psychotic changes. Its duration may be prolonged and in some the mental symptoms may precede the more specific symptoms of an attack. Some have argued that this is more common in familial hemiplegic migraine than in sporadic cases (Fenichel, 1985), although agreement on this point does not exist.

As already indicated, in the majority of patients the hemisyndrome constitutes the major part of the migrainous aura and symptoms rapidly resolve to be replaced by a headache. This group appears to be generally benign and carries a favourable prognosis. It has been customary for some to refer to this group as 'Type I'. This is in contrast to the less common but more troublesome group referred to as 'Type II', in which the hemiparetic symptoms and/or aphasia continue in and through the headache phase of an attack (Whitty, 1953). In some that are generally grouped in the second category a biphasic presentation may occur with an initial resolution of the hemisyndrome, only for it to return later on in the same attack. It is in this second group that the duration of symptoms is longer and measured in hours not minutes and occasionally in days.

Inevitably persistence of signs much beyond 24 h brings up the question of infarction, which is rare during migraine, but well recognized. Most reports are of cerebral infarction during the course of an attack of headache with nausea and vomiting, in a known migraine subject, usually adult (Cohen and Taylor, 1979; Spaccavento and Solomon, 1984). Cerebral infarction in a child with migraine is very rare. In their review of 40 children with 'complicated migraine' (virtually all with unilateral symptoms/signs), Rossi *et al.* (1980) observed no instance of permanent neurological sequelae reflecting infarction in the 25 who were followed for from 1 to 15 years. Ment *et al.* (1980), however, reported three children with hemiplegic migraine, in whom permanent neurological deficit occurred. The subject is well discussed by Barlow (1984).

Nausea and vomiting are common with hemiplegic attacks of whatever type, but generally this is a less striking feature than in other forms of migraine (Whitty, 1986).

Differential diagnosis

The above onset of symptoms inevitably raises the question of the diagnosis of a neurological disorder other than migraine, particularly when there is no family history of migraine and no history suggestive of previous migrainous attacks in the patient. Such a situation may exist in up to 50% of children when they first present (Rossi *et al.*, 1980).

While a headache frequently accompanies the hemisyndrome it may not be a prominent symptom within the attack and occasionally it may be absent. Even when headache is present alternative diagnoses still have to be considered and appropriate investigations carried out. Differentiating an attack of hemiplegic migraine from a focal seizure with a Todd's paralysis may be difficult, particularly when attempting retrospective evaluation of the nature of attacks. With a migrainous episode headache is common, the 'march' or progression of the hemiparesis is longer than with a Todd's paralysis, and any period of paraesthesia will last typically for much longer than in a Todd's paralysis. Clonic movements in migraine are an extreme rarity. While nausea (and vomiting) is less common in hemiplegic than in other forms of migraine, its presence with or without visual phenomena will lend strong support to the diagnosis of migraine. As reported by Rossi *et al.* (1980) differing sides may be affected in different attacks and shifts of side may even be seen occasionally in a single attack.

For the clinician perhaps the most worrying differential is from a vascular malformation or a tumour – particularly an arteriovenous malformation. There is very little information on the specific incidence of vascular anomalies in children who are having attacks analogous to hemiplegic migraine. In adults the incidence is very low. Arteriovenous malformations are more probable if epilepsy or a prolonged disturbance of consciousness occurs or if the hemiparesis lasts for more than a few hours. Nevertheless, it is recognized that both disturbed consciousness and a hemiparesis may persist for considerable periods of time in migraine.

Vascular disease – vasculitis, fibromuscular disease, occlusive disease and embolic disease – may produce hemiparetic attacks. Vasculitis or an 'arteritis' may occur with hemiparetic symptoms in conjunction with a systemic disorder such as lupus erythematosis or polyarteritis nodosa. However, both situations are rare and in the majority there will be evidence of more widespread systemic disease, but this is not inevitable. Occlusive vascular disease may occur from a variety of mechanisms and causations. Many will be secondary to arteritic or thrombophlebitic disease that gives rise to thrombosis. Overall, pyogenic meningitis and particularly tuberculous meningitis together are the commonest causes of thrombotic disease. Although diagnostic difficulties seldom occur in such a situation, very occasionally with tuberculous meningitis the underlying infection may not at first be obvious. Cerebral thrombosis is well documented as a consequence of sickle cell disease and the end-result may well be a hemiparesis. Trauma to the neck or the tonsillar fossa may induce thrombosis and a hemiparesis (Bickerstaff, 1964a). The late effects of radiotherapy can give rise to small arterial occlusions and a hemiparesis with other associated symptoms. Cyanotic heart disease carries with it a risk of embolization and thrombosis with an allied risk of cerebral abscess (Clarkson *et al.*, 1967).

Recurrent occlusive vascular disease is typical of Moyamoya disease. While 90% of cases that have been reported have been in Japanese subjects with a predominance of females, a substantial number of non-Japanese cases have now appeared in the literature. Moyamoya disease may present in two ways: either as cerebral ischaemia in children or SAH in adults (Levin, 1982). Maki and colleagues (1976) classified the clinical presentation of their 24 cases as 'transient ischaemic episodes' with residual neurological deficit (five cases); ischaemic episodes with residual neurological deficit – hemiparesis, aphasia or visual field deficits (12 cases); sudden onset episodes with little or no recovery, including SAH (five cases); and a miscellaneous group of two cases, one of which presented with seizures and the other which had macrocephaly only. Hemiparesis which may be alternating is the most common finding among children. Facial palsy, nystagmus, aphasia, dysarthria, pseudobulbar palsy, involuntary movements and seizures have all been described. High definition CT scanning may support the diagnosis, but the diagnosis still rests principally on cerebral angiography. In all cases there is occlusion of the supraclinoid part of both internal carotid arteries, with dilated collaterals in the basal ganglia, and leptomeningeal and transdural collateral anastomosis – the hazy smoke appearance for which the Japanese word is 'Moyamoya'.

A miscellaneous group of abnormalities of the blood vessels has been associated with childhood thrombosis; these have ranged from agenesis or hypoplasia to 'kinks and coils' of the vessels. One entity which seems much more common in the older female is that of fibromuscular dysplasia in which the angiographic appearances are of a string of beads. In a third of such patients (Mettinger and Ericson, 1982) unilateral throbbing headaches occur prior to infarction. It is speculated by some that taking the contraceptive pill may precipitate thrombotic episodes in young women with this underlying abnormality.

In the management of children with leukaemia there is a question about whether the focal neurological deficits that may occur are due to chemotherapeutic agents, or to radiation therapy. L-Asparaginase has been associated with a small incidence of haemorrhagic infarction probably related to changes in blood coagulation factors (Cairo *et al.*, 1980).

A metabolic basis for occlusive disease may exist in some. In homocystinuria, particularly after any surgical procedure, there may be a risk of thrombosis and this may include the cerebral vasculature. In the presence of a history of recurrent attacks, particularly if these are in an individual with Marfan-like features present, homocystinuria has to be considered. Hypercholesterolaemia may first present clinically with occlusive disease affecting the cerebral vasculature. The MELAS syndrome (Mitochondrial myopathy, Encephalopathy, Lactic Acidosis, and Stroke-like episodes) is referred to elsewhere (see Chapters 1 and 6).

It has to be remembered that with any of the specific differential diagnoses referred to above migraine may also occur in the same individual. Therefore, this demands a careful evaluation with the support of relevant investigations in any individual in whom a focal neurological deficit occurs, even if a diagnosis of migraine has been confidently established.

Investigations

In the absence of a clear history of previous migraine attacks, and whether or not there is a family history, in virtually all instances clinicians faced with a child with a hemiparesis (with or without headache or alteration in consciousness) will want to consider relevant investigations. In practice CT scanning, usually high resolution, will be available and many would regard this as being a 'central investigation'. Certainly any patient with a hemiparesis persisting for more than a few days warrants investigation. Similarly, persistence of symptoms or signs between attacks, and frank epilepsy with attacks, raise the question of a structural lesion such as an arteriovenous malformation or a tumour. With the rare event of SAH due either to a bleed from an arteriovenous malformation or a congenital berry aneurysm, the sudden onset of severe and persisting headache often with nuchal rigidity leaves little doubt about the need for further investigation – CT scanning, CSF examination and, usually, angiography.

The range of vascular anomalies in childhood extends beyond arteriovenous malformations alone. Arteritic lesions may occur, fibromuscular dysplasia particularly in females and simple kinks in major blood vessels may result in specific attacks. For this reason in the presence of a persistent neurological deficit and a negative CT scan, cerebral angiography must be considered. However, alongside this must be considered the dangers of such investigations. It is well documented that angiography performed during the course of a migrainous episode may exacerbate the attack and leave a permanent deficit (Lai et al., 1982). Between attacks it is equally well documented that angiography can precipitate attacks which may again be severe with a persistent deficit (Blau and Whitty, 1955; Bradshaw and Parsons, 1965), although with modern contrast materials, and techniques such as digital subtraction angiography, risks are now considered remote.

CSF examination is necessary if bleeding is suspected or if there is a suspicion of infection. The presence of xanthochromia with or without frankly blood-stained CSF strongly suggests the diagnosis of a bleed. However, the CSF may be abnormal in the acute stage of hemiplegic migraine. Mild elevations of protein have been reported from several studies and a few patients have had increased cell counts, typically lymphocytic (Kremenitzer and Golden, 1974; Rossi et al., 1985).

Electroencephalography is considered by many to be unhelpful (Whitty, 1986). Diffuse or focal slowing is the most common findings between attacks (Rossi et al., 1980). During attacks lateralized slowing may be found over the appropriate hemisphere but perversely the abnormality can be generalized or localized to the 'wrong' side.

Jensen et al. (1981b) studied cerebral blood flow in four female members of a family with hemiplegic migraine using xenon-133 inhalation during and between attacks. Their findings suggested a lower flow over the appropriate hemisphere during attacks but normal flow between attacks. Hosking et al. (1978) had similar findings in a girl with alternating hemiplegia.

The range of investigations will, of course, be dictated by the clinical picture in the individual child, and in many with a clear-cut history of recurrent migrainous attacks, complex or common, together with a positive family history, it is very reasonable to embark upon none.

Outlook

In a high proportion of children with hemiplegic migraine the frequency and severity of attacks decrease with age. The attacks, however, are often replaced by other forms of migraine.

In spite of the frequency of attacks the majority with the so-called 'Type I' attacks have a benign outlook (Rossi *et al.*, 1980; Jensen *et al.*, 1981a). In those with the less common Type II attacks a small but significant risk exists for a permanent focal deficit together with, in some very rare instances, intellectual deterioration (Ment *et al.*, 1980).

Basilar artery migraine

The constellation of symptoms and signs that go to make up the entity of BAM are those that are related to the tissue supplied by the basilar–vertebral system. They will thus include a complex of cranial nerve, posterior cerebral hemisphere, cerebellar and corticospinal signs that will vary greatly from patient to patient.

In the definitive report that established the entity of 'basilar artery' migraine Bickerstaff (1961a) suggested that occurrence was most typically in adolescent and preadolescent females.

Because of the very great variation between individuals in the extent of symptoms and attacks Lapkin and Golden (1978) suggested a division of patients into three groups:

Group I: Episodic headache and/or a strong family history of migraine and one transient recurrent neurological symptom referrable to the basilar–vertebral arterial tree.
Group II: Episodic headache and/or a strong family history of migraine and two transient recurrent neurological symptoms referrable to the basilar–vertebral arterial tree.
Group III: Episodic headache and/or a strong family history of migraine and three or more recurrent neurological symptoms referrable to the basilar–vertebral arterial tree.

It is recognized that with many migraine attacks there will be some symptoms that are, or could be, attributable to the basilar artery territory, and therefore in practice it is only the Group III of Lapkin and Golden that is most usually designated as BAM. However, there is variation, and estimations of incidence from published reports depend largely on the definition used. Thus, while Barlow (1984) found an incidence of vertigo of 19% in his series of patients with migraine, he only found 2.3% when a more restricted definition was employed. Somewhat by contrast Hockaday (1979) noted that 24% in a series of 122 children with migraine had focal disturbances referrable to the basilar artery distribution, with a further 15% as 'possibles'. Brown (1977) and Lapkin and Golden (1978) have in addition expressed opinions that BAM in childhood is not rare.

While Bickerstaff (1961a) stressed the usual frequency in girls in later childhood and adolescence, others have suggested that the onset may be in infancy and that the sex distribution at least in younger children was probably roughly equal (Lapkin and Golden, 1978) or even more common in boys (Hockaday, 1979). The difficulties of making a diagnosis in young children is real when this depends so much upon description of subjective symptoms.

Barlow (1984) summarized the issue as follows in regard to patients with three or more symptoms referrable to the basilar artery territory:

1. Age of onset can range from infancy to middle adult years.
2. Strong female predominance from puberty onwards.
3. Lower female bias in the younger prepubertal patients, who are also less likely to have evidence of headache as an index clue to the migrainic nature of their disorder.

While Barlow (1984) suggested that familial recurrence of fully developed BAM was rare, Sturzenegger and Meienberg (1985) in their study of 82 adolescent or adult patients with BAM found a 73% incidence of positive family histories of migraine, 75% of whom were on the female side. Golden and French (1975) in a study of eight children found a positive family history of migraine in seven and in six more than one family member was affected. The seven patients with a positive family history had a total of 16 affected relatives, 14 on the maternal side of the family, with 15 of the 16 being female. Lapkin and Golden (1978) found an incidence of 86% positive family histories in their patients, again predominantly on the maternal side of the family and female. However, these publications have not provided details of the type of migraine that occurred in family members so Barlow's suggestion of the rarity of fully developed BAM in family members may hold true.

Clinical features

There is enormous variability in the clinical presentation of BAM, although within individuals it is common for the clinical presentation to be similar. However, diagnosis depends upon the occurrence of symptoms and signs of multiple cranial nerve dysfunction in conjunction with ataxia and weakness due to corticospinal involvement. In most but not all children, the specific neurological symptoms and signs precede headache, which may only occur as specific features of the attack resolve. Although Hockaday (1979) noted headache in all her cases with BAM, both Golden and French (1975) and Lapkin and Golden (1978) noted a small number in whom the symptom of headache was denied. In only five out of Hockaday's 29 children was the headache occipital in location.

It is argued that visual symptoms are common in children with BAM and they are often the first specific neurological symptom to occur in an attack (Bickerstaff, 1986). Hockaday (1979) would only accept visual symptoms as indicative of basilar system involvement if both half fields of vision were involved. The symptoms may include tunnel vision, total amblyopia and positive or negative hallucinations. Bickerstaff (1962) has argued that if there are positive phenomena they are likely to consist of 'flashes or blobs of light'. Ataxia is probably the next of the specific symptoms to appear, often accompanied by vertigo and sometimes tinnitus. Dysarthria as distinct from dysphasia is common and may with the other clinical features of an attack suggest intoxication by drugs or alcohol in an older child. In those children able to describe the symptoms numbness and tingling around the face, mouth and tongue, and in the hands and feet – bilaterally – is common, occurring typically early in an attack.

The range of other symptoms and signs that may occur in BAM are all those that may be expected when dysfunction occurs in the basilar artery territory. These may include nystagmus, diplopia, third nerve and seventh nerve lesions and internuclear ophthalmoplegia and pyramidal dysfunction. The occurrence of these further specific features tends to be associated with the more severe and prolonged attacks, a number of which have their specific neurological phenomena after rather than before the headache.

While Lapkin and Golden (1978) felt that nausea/vomiting was rare most other authors have found it to be common and prostrating (Hockaday, 1979; Bickerstaff, 1986), and often associated with pallor. Lethargy and drowsiness are very common during attacks. This may extend to coma. Very often this is most noticeable as specific symptoms recede but may occur earlier (Bickerstaff, 1961b). Prolonged impairment of consciousness, however, demands further examination and evaluation of the diagnosis. Drop attacks sometimes resulting in injury may occur as part of a BAM attack, often simply reflecting loss of postural control and if there is loss of consciousness it is only transient.

An association between BAM and epilepsy has been of interest for some time (Basser, 1969). Camfield et al. (1978) described four adolescents who had BAM, infrequent seizures and severe EEG changes. They were otherwise well. The infrequent seizures usually followed a migrainous aura and were easily controlled with anticonvulsant medication. Swanson and Vick (1978) reported the EEG findings during the course of a BAM attack and this was typical of a photoconvulsive response. They reported a favourable response to anticonvulsant medication. Panayiotopoulos (1980) described a 14-year-old boy with attacks reminiscent of BAM and an EEG showing continuous spike and slow wave activity confined to the posterior region and inhibited by eye opening but retained when in darkness. His attacks ceased with anticonvulsant medication. The author questioned, therefore, whether the syndrome in his patient was migrainous or epileptic. While Lapkin et al. (1977) suggested that transient functional disturbance of the brainstem can produce EEG changes, Bickerstaff (1986) considered it just as likely that the EEG changes and seizures were caused by the effects of transient ischaemia on a potentially epileptic brain. For fuller discussion see Chapter 7.

Finally, it is important to state that although the severity of attacks can vary, the specific symptoms of BAM rarely last more than an hour, and are then followed in most cases by headache with or without nausea, and often drowsiness and sleep.

Differential diagnosis

In the presence of a positive family history and a history of recurrent and transient brainstem dysfunction in conjunction with a headache there is seldom diagnostic difficulty. However, in the absence of a positive family history for migraine, or of a past history in the child of migrainous episodes and faced with a longer than usual attack, consideration has to be given to alternative diagnoses.

Vertebrobasilar insufficiency is rare in childhood (Mori et al., 1979). The existence of a Blalock–Taussig anastomosis for congenital heart disease (Clarkson et al., 1967) may, however, be associated with basilar insufficiency. Congenital malformations of the base of the brain – abnormalities of the odontoid, platybasia and basilar impression and the Chiari malformation – may give rise to transient neurological symptoms of brainstem dysfunction.

Posterior fossa tumours present with an evolving and (sometimes intermittently) progressive picture and, with the exception of an infiltrating lesion of the brainstem, will usually be associated with symptoms and signs of raised intracranial pressure. Hamartomatous lesions in the brainstem may produce an intermittent picture of brainstem dysfunction, but this is more reminiscent of multiple sclerosis (itself rare in childhood) than of migraine (Abroms et al., 1971; Duquette et al., 1987). Several metabolic disorders may simulate attacks similar to BAM. Homocystinuria, pyruvate carboxylase deficiency, ornithine transcarbamylase deficiency and some organic acidaemias may produce attacks reminiscent of BAM. However in most there is evidence of persisting neurological dysfunction between attacks. Sturzenegger and Meienberg (1985) have argued that the most important differential diagnoses to BAM are temporal lobe epilepsy, hysterical attacks and vertebral–basilar insufficiency. In the case of temporal lobe epilepsy, while it is acknowledged that at times the distinction may be difficult, headaches, visual hallucinations and staggering are much more typical of migraine than they are of epilepsy.

Investigations

With a clear history specific investigations are seldom indicated. If such a history is lacking then structural abnormalities must be excluded by appropriate neurological investigation. CT scanning is usually adequate.

The possibility of a metabolic basis will require appropriate investigations.

The EEG in most series has been normal between attacks. During attacks paroxysmal slow-wave activity with occipital predominance, although not specific, is a common finding (see Chapter 7).

Testing of vestibular function (Eviatar, 1981) has revealed a high incidence of abnormalities in children with BAM and this appears to correlate with the severity of attacks.

The CSF, as in some patients with hemiplegic migraine during attacks, may show a lymphocytic pleocytosis and mildly elevated protein.

Outlook

The outlook for most children with BAM is good. Many will have attacks of common or classical migraine interspersed with their complex attacks and later evolve to have these forms of attacks alone. Hockaday (1979) has nevertheless reported a poor outcome in two of her patients in whom the attacks were of very early onset (in infancy).

Ophthalmoplegic migraine

Some of the earliest accounts of ophthalmoplegic migraine extend back into the nineteenth century. In spite of this, however, this form of special migraine is rare and probably the least common of all complex migraines (Barlow, 1984). This author has only encountered one case in 10 years and other published series testify to its rarity (Friedman et al., 1962b; Pearce and Foster, 1965). Besides this some of the earlier accounts did not, because of their absence of definitive investigations, necessarily distinguish ophthalmoplegic migraine from symptoms and signs due for example to an aneurysm on the Circle of Willis.

As with most forms of migraine a positive family history is likely, but may not be as common as with others (Walsh and Hoyt, 1969).

Clinical features

Ophthalmoplegic migraine is in effect an isolated lesion of the third nerve, although very occasionally there may be involvement of the fourth and fifth nerves. The downward and outward position, the ptosis, diplopia on passive lifting of the eyelid are characteristic and in most cases there is dilatation of the pupil. Pain around the eye or on the ipsilateral temple side is usual and, together with head tilt, for most completes the clinical presentation. Somewhat in contrast to hemiplegic migraine the focal deficit tends to follow rather than precede the headache or retro-orbital pain (Friedman et al., 1962b).

An early age of onset is characteristic. Bickerstaff (1964b) has suggested the first attack is almost always before 12 years of age and accounts exist of its occurrence in infants at and below the age of 12 months (Robertson and Schnitzler, 1978; Durkan et al., 1981; Woody and Blaw, 1986). Attacks will typically commence with headache and often be accompanied by blurred vision or diplopia. However, the more specific features of ophthalmoplegia tend to follow these prodromal symptoms and may follow on after the headache.

The headache itself may be typically migrainous, although, in contrast with classical or hemiplegic migraine, it is invariably ipsilateral. Anorexia and vomiting may occur; the latter often marks the termination of an individual attack. Not only may the ophthalmoplegia typically occur after the headache has subsided but it may also follow on hours afterwards. When pain does accompany the ophthalmoplegia, then it is typically retro-orbital. However, it would appear that in infants or young children this pain is usually insignificant because of short duration or mild nature.

The duration of the ophthalmoplegia is very variable, ranging from hours up to months. In the majority of cases complete recovery does take place, although often with repeated and severe attacks residual dysfunction may result. The frequency of attacks is clearly variable. Several reports describe repeated similar attacks. Many suggest a wide interval between attacks, but all with sufficient follow-up indicate that migrainous attacks of the classic type occur later, in most cases irrespective of the recurrence of ophthalmoplegic attacks.

Differential diagnosis

The differential diagnosis at the time of the first attack is wide. Some alternative diagnoses are relatively easy to make or exclude, others less so.

A congenital berry aneurysm can produce a clinical picture to all intents and purposes identical to that of ophthalmoplegic migraine. Such an aneurysm would be either of the posterior communicating artery or the supraclinoid portion of the internal carotid artery. With an aneurysm, however, it is more common for the ophthalmoplegia to precede the pain, for there to be trigeminal nerve signs and for the pain to have a neuralgic character rather than the throbbing quality more typical of migraine.

In recognition of the overlapping symptoms between a berry aneurysm and ophthalmoplegic migraine, Walsh and O'Doherty (1960) suggested the following diagnostic criteria for ophthalmoplegic migraine:

1. A history of typical migraine headache with crescendo quality.

2. Ophthalmoplegia, including one or more nerves and possibly alternating sides with attacks, the paralysis usually appearing subsequent to an established migraine pattern.
3. Exclusion of other causes by arteriography, surgery or autopsy.

Many will accept these criteria, certainly when applied to adults, but the need for arteriography in children may be questioned.

Cerebral aneurysms are exceedingly uncommon in children. Matson (1965) found only three cases under the age of 5 years, all presented with symptoms of SAH and none with ophthalmoplegia. Patel and Richardson (1971) reported similar findings. Probably the only reported case of ophthalmoplegia caused by an aneurysm in a child under 10 years was that of Thompson and Pribram (1969). Their patient aged 1 month had a right internal carotid berry aneurysm and the presentation was with bilateral ophthalmoplegia and lethargy. In addition there was a quadriplegia and evidence of hydrocephalus. Their review of the literature suggested that under the age of 2 years aneurysms present with either hydrocephalus or the signs of SAH. No reports appear to exist of children under the age of 10 years with an aneurysm that presents with an ophthalmoplegia in the absence of the signs of SAH. From these reports it could be argued that the most basic point that distinguishes between ophthalmoplegic migraine and an aneurysm is age. Ophthalmoplegic migraine is far more likely to be the diagnosis when onset is in childhood, with the opposite being the case in adulthood.

Intracranial tumour must always be considered in a child presenting with an ophthalmoplegia. Infiltrating brainstem gliomas may present with an ophthalmo-plegia as the only neurological abnormality, although more often than not there will be other cranial nerve lesions on both sides of the midline as well as corticospinal or cerebellar signs. As well as this, headache is seldom significant and may indeed be absent. Progression of headache or physical signs makes confusion with migraine unlikely. Extrinsic tumours such as leukaemic infiltration or tumours of bone may produce diagnostic difficulties.

Head trauma is a frequent cause of ophthalmoplegia in the young, but the history and the relationship to the trauma is usually such that confusion with migraine seldom occurs.

Chronic sinusitis with a mucocele of the sphenoid sinus may be associated with periodic headaches and recurrent third nerve palsies. In some the history of headache may extend over several years and in most the history of chronic sinus disease is obvious. Infection and inflammation, besides that involving the paranasal sinuses, may produce a third nerve palsy. Tuberculous meningitis as a granulomatous basilar meningitis may produce an ophthalmoplegia, although because of the more generalized meningeal and systemic signs diagnosis does not usually present difficulties. Diphtheria, tetanus, viral hepatitis, mumps and tick paralysis have all been reported to produce a third nerve lesion. But here again the other features of these infections seldom if ever produce diagnostic confusion with migraine.

Ischaemic infarction of the third nerve, usually associated with diabetes mellitus is the most common cause of a third nerve lesion in adults. In children it is unknown, except very occasionally in children with longstanding juvenile diabetes.

Myasthenia gravis, which may present with ptosis, bears only the most superficial resemblance to a third nerve palsy. Bilaterality of some degree is usual, and weakness of facial expression, diplopia not consistent with a third nerve lesion, and a normal pupil, suffice to distinguish this from migraine. If doubt persists the response to intravenous edrophonium chloride should remove it.

The Tolosa–Hunt syndrome of painful ophthalmoplegia typically reported in adults, only rarely in children (Terrence and Samaha, 1973), has features that overlap those of ophthalmoplegic migraine. In the Tolosa–Hunt syndrome pain and ophthalmoplegia occur simultaneously and generally the time-course is longer than in migraine. Nevertheless, Kandt and Goldstein (1985) described a 6-year-old girl in whom the features of both situations undoubtedly overlapped and gave rise to diagnostic uncertainty. As they pointed out, Hunt *et al.* (1961) gave six criteria for the diagnosis of the Tolosa–Hunt syndrome: steady pain behind the eye, often gnawing or 'boring'; involvement of nerves passing through the cavernous sinus; symptoms for days or weeks; spontaneous remission, sometimes with residual deficits; attacks at intervals of months or years; and exhaustive studies excluding involvement outside the cavernous sinus. In 1976 Hunt added a seventh criterion, steroid responsiveness (Hunt, 1976). An elevation of the ESR is common and the supposed underlying mechanism is that of an idiopathic granulomatous inflammation of the cavernous sinus.

In a comprehensive review of the literature on ophthalmoplegic migraine Kandt and Goldstein (1985) argue that in many cases the criteria for diagnosis of ophthalmoplegic migraine suggested by Walsh and O'Doherty (1960) were in fact absent, and that the possibility of Tolosa–Hunt syndrome existed in many. The therapeutic implications of the findings are concerned with whether steroids should be employed in *suspected* ophthalmoplegic migraine at least until the diagnosis is certain and other causes of ophthalmoplegia have been excluded.

Investigations

In any child presenting with a third nerve lesion, without a history of an obvious cause for the clinical features that render diagnosis certain, the principal question has to be which neuroradiological studies should be undertaken.

Unlike the situation with adults, most aneurysms in children are quite large. With modern CT scanning it would seem reasonable to embark upon this investigation and not submit a child to angiography unless there is a very specific indication (Bailey *et al.*, 1984). However, in a child with a history that is highly suggestive of ophthalmoplegic migraine, the known rarity of aneurysms presenting in the absence of any evidence of bleeding does beg the question whether even CT scanning is necessary, although most would consider it advisable.

Outlook

The frequency of attacks in any individual with ophthalmoplegic migraine is variable and unpredictable. The most common pattern is that there are recurrent attacks at widely spaced intervals, although in some patients frequent attacks do occur. The long-term outlook is also uncertain. In the majority of patients uncomplicated migraine attacks occur in addition to ophthalmoplegic attacks and ultimately continue as the only form of migraine. However, even in those patients whose attacks ultimately cease, there may be concern, because the ophthalmoplegia may remit only partially, or not at all (Van Pelt and Andermann, 1964; Robertson and Schnitzler, 1978; Durkan *et al.*, 1981). An unresolved question is whether steroid therapy should be actively considered in every child presenting with 'painful ophthalmoplegia' (Kandt and Goldstein, 1985), because of the difficulty that lies in distinguishing Tolosa–Hunt syndrome from ophthalmoplegic migraine.

Confusional migraine, Alice in Wonderland syndrome, migraine stupor, transient global amnesia

There are some forms of migraine in which the predominant features may be alteration in consciousness and disordered thought processes. These are confusional migraine, Alice in Wonderland syndrome, migraine stupor and transient global amnesia. While these four forms of migraine attacks have some overlap in the phenomena observed during attacks, they are for the most part sufficiently distinct for them to be considered individually, as below. However, it is recognized that mental changes also occur in other forms of migraine, for example in hemiplegic migraine (Bradshaw and Parsons, 1965; Lai et al., 1982; Fenichel, 1985) and BAM (Bickerstaff, 1961b; Swanson and Vick, 1978).

Confusional migraine

The frequency of a confusional state as the principal manifestation of migraine is difficult to estimate. Gascon and Barlow (1970) described four patients, three boys and one girl ranging in age from 8 to 16 years at presentation, who presented with attacks of acute confusion. Ehyai and Fenichel (1978) described a 5% incidence in a series of 100 patients of acute confusional states and Barlow (1984) found a similar percentage in a series of 300, in three of whom amnesia was more prominent than the confusion. Fourteen of his 15 patients were boys between 8 and 16 years of age.

In all published reports there is a greater frequency of acute confusional migraine in boys than girls. In part this is undoubtedly due to a number of episodes being induced or precipitated by trauma in sport (Emery, 1977), but even without the factor of trauma (often minor) the frequency remains higher in boys than girls. In virtually all reported cases the history includes an account of common or classical migraine (Gascon and Barlow, 1970; Emery, 1977).

Clinical features
Headache is often an insignificant aspect of attacks, being either trivial or absent. The confusional symptoms are either the first evidence of an attack or follow after a headache is established, Crowell et al. (1984) and Gascon and Barlow (1970) comment on the relatively rapid evolution of the initial phenomena, with the confusional state as a relatively late phenomenon during a total attack. The headache itself may be preceded by an aura, be unilateral and be accompanied by symptoms such as dizziness, eye symptoms, nausea and vomiting. In many it may not be until recovery that a history can be obtained of migraine symptoms, either with the attack or on previous occasions.

The confusional state itself is very often characterized by inattention, distractability, and difficulties in maintaining continuous speech or other activities. Agitation and disturbances in memory are common. In a number of patients (Brott and Leviton, 1976) agitation may be severe and associated with violent behaviour. Language production remains intact and obscene utterances are common (Gascon and Barlow, 1970). Tremulousness and fear occur in some. Some will pass into a stupor (see below).

Haas *et al.* (1975) and Emery (1977) have drawn attention to minor head trauma as a trigger for attacks. In some of these individuals there may be a gap of between 30 and 60 min between the trauma and the onset of confusional symptoms, making post-traumatic concussion unlikely. The duration of confusional symptoms may be as short as 10 min or as long as 2 days. A typical duration will be between 6 and 8 h. Fluctuation in symptoms in an attack is common and usually an attack will be terminated by sleep (Tinuper *et al.*, 1985; Parrino *et al.*, 1986).

The frequency of attacks seems to be low in any individual and in a number of patients single episodes only are recorded.

Alice in Wonderland syndrome

While in acute confusional migraine an assumption can be made that cerebral dysfunction is diffuse, there are some children in whom more specific alterations in mental status occur. These may include perceptual abnormalities, distortions of body image, and alterations in subjective time sense (Lippman, 1952). Todd (1955) described what Lippman has referred to as the 'syndrome of Alice in Wonderland' in six adult patients. The employment of this name arose from the knowledge that Lewis Carroll suffered from migraine and that the experiences of Alice were in part a reflection of the varying perceptual abnormalities that Carroll had undoubtedly experienced in attacks of migraine. Golden described the syndrome in two children, a boy and a girl both aged 11 years (Golden, 1979).

Clinical features
Family histories of migraine are common and most patients themselves have histories of headaches. Attacks typically occur as a prodrome but at times this may be several days before a headache (Lippman, 1952), and in some instances headaches do not occur. In others symptoms referrable to basilar artery dysfunction, such as ataxia and vertigo, occur with the perceptual abnormalities.

Sacks (1970) has defined five important categories of dysfunction typical of the Alice in Wonderland syndrome:

1. Complex disorders of visual perception (conveniently described as Lilliputian, Brobdignagian, zoom, mosaic and cinematographic vision, etc.).
2. Complex difficulties in the perception and use of the body (apraxia and agnosia).
3. Speech and language disorders.
4. States of double or multiple consciousness, often associated with feelings of *déjà vu* or *jamais vu* and other disorders and dislocations of time perception.
5. Elaborate dreamy, nightmarish, trance-like or delirious states.

Migraine stupor

Lee and Lance (1977) described seven patients between 10 and 52 years of age with stupor lasting 2 h to 5 days during attacks of migraine. In four of the seven patients the attacks started with confusion, aggression or hysteria, five had an homonymous hemianopia, and six suffered from ataxia, incoordination and dysarthria. Four noted paraesthesiae and three had a dilated pupil during attacks. A variety of alternative diagnoses to migraine were considered and excluded. Therefore, from this study it can be argued that when stupor occurs it is very often in association with brainstem signs suggesting a primary involvement of the basilar–vertebral system. The authors speculate that if a single site is to be implicated in migraine stupor it may be the mid brain because it is the origin of the reticular activating system and because of the dilatation of the pupil.

Transient global amnesia

It has been argued by Barlow (1984) that distinguishing TGA when referring to confusional migraine would confer little advantage. Nevertheless, others (e.g. Bruyn, 1986) have argued for its separate consideration in migraine, although typically in adults of middle years and the elderly (Olivarius and Jensen, 1979). In this it differs from acute confusional migraine which seems to concentrate in the early teenage years. It has however been well described in childhood (Jensen, 1980).

Clinical features

Olivarius and Jensen (1979) described typical episodes of TGA as starting abruptly, often precipitated by mental or physical stress. Consciousness remains unaltered but the patient is confused and disorientated with perseveration of thought, speech and behaviour. Routine actions may be undertaken but the patient shows evidence of loss of memory, usually repeating the same question over and over again. The patient is unable to store new information, has a relative loss of memory for recent events and a retrograde amnesia for a variable duration.

Duration typically is for minutes to hours and ends with a gradual return of intact memory function. While the retrograde amnesia diminishes with time, amnesia for the attack itself persists. Single, or in some patients two or three, episodes is the usual pattern.

Differential diagnosis

Confusional migraine and Alice in Wonderland syndrome

Probably the principal alternative diagnosis to acute confusional migraine is a toxic-metabolic encephalopathy. Barlow (1984) suggests that intoxication with drugs, either accidently ingested or for thrills, is much more likely to be the cause of an acute confusional state than migraine. With this he urges a careful scrutiny with a combination of the usual 'toxic screen' and a history of available drugs (including those from illicit sources) being undertaken.

Metabolic derangements, as in the early stages of Reye's syndrome or due to inborn errors of urea, amino acid and organic acid metabolism, where symptoms may be intermittent, must also be considered. Severe migraine with encephalopathy may also occur with mitochondrial abnormalities (Dvorkin et al., 1987). Gascon and Barlow (1970) mention hypoglycaemic encephalopathy and water intoxication as being among the possible differential diagnoses.

Viral encephalitis may present with confusion and agitation, without fever or other signs of CNS infection or inflammation. Such a differentiation may be difficult when it is recognized that CSF protein may be elevated, and a pleocytosis be present, in juvenile migraine. Fever may also occur with migraine attacks although it is rarely persistent. Prolonged episodes and persistent fever would, however, on clinical grounds support the diagnosis of an encephalitis rather than migraine. Differentiation from a seizure disorder may sometimes prove difficult. No major difficulty should be encountered in distinguishing between acute confusional migraine and a postictal confusional state because it is improbable that in the latter there would not be a clear history of a preceding seizure. However, in the case of minor or temporal lobe status epilepticus it may be difficult to distinguish from migraine confusion on clinical grounds. Nevertheless, in most there will be a history of a pre-existing seizure disorder and certainly EEG examination will serve to distinguish easily between the two situations.

There are acute psychogenic states that may bear a superficial resemblance to acute confusional migraine. These may be an acute schizophrenic reaction, acute panic attacks, or acute mania. While agitation is a feature, as in acute confusional migraine, orientation and intellectual functioning including memory and attention are better preserved in psychogenic states. Besides this, with psychogenic causes the onset is generally more gradual.

Migraine stupor
The differential diagnosis of migraine stupor is similar to that of acute confusional migraine and the Alice in Wonderland syndrome. The possibilities of metabolic disturbance due to ornithine transcarbamylase deficiency and other causes of hyperammonaemia should be considered (Russell, 1973; Rowe *et al.*, 1986).

Transient global amnesia
Three disorders which may give rise to amnesic episodes are epilepsy, migraine and hysteria. In complex partial seizures memory loss as an isolated phenomenon would be very rare. Other symptoms such as an aura and automatisms are typically present in complex partial seizures.

Investigations

In a child with a picture either of acute confusional migraine, or migraine stupor or the Alice in Wonderland syndrome metabolic investigations are crucial. In the case of toxins or drugs it has to be recognized that most 'toxic screens' are not wholly comprehensive and diligent history taking is vital. Electroencephalography will enable a distinction to be made between migraine, confusional stupor and minor status epilepticus and assists with the diagnosis of an encephalitic condition (Tinuper *et al.*, 1985).

Envoi

Special forms (variants) of migraine, or complicated migraine, whichever term is preferred, have been recognized and described in childhood for many years. However, with the continual expansion of literature on these syndromes, some clinical overlap between different varieties is recognized and further examples emerge. Their delineation as 'multiple syndromes' is helpful mainly in considering their differential diagnosis.

Summary

Bruyn (1986) suggests that 'the notions of common migraine (migraena vulgaris), classical migraine (migraenus ophthalmica), ophthalmoplegic, basilar and (familial) hemiplegic migraine have earned their citizen rights long ago'.

This chapter looks at the principal forms of complicated migraine occurring in childhood. Their occurrence always raises questions in the mind of the clinician about whether they are migrainous or whether, because of the focal neurological symptoms, there is an alternative diagnosis. So much will depend upon the history – of the attack in question and of any previous attacks in the patient – and the family history.

In hemiplegic migraine there may be a family history of similar attacks, typically on the maternal side, or at least a strong family history of migraine. Hemiplegia typically occurs as part of the prodrome and may very often be accompanied by altered consciousness. Visual symptoms are also present in many, indicating involvement of the posterior cerebral hemisphere. Differentiation from a postictal Todd's paralysis is necessary and should not be difficult with a clear history, but differentiation from some other vascular events can be difficult and in many will necessitate definitive further investigations. Angiography should, however, be used with caution, because of the risks of increasing the patient's neurological deficit. In general the outlook is favourable in children with hemiplegic migraine, with attacks decreasing in frequency with age. However, many will go on to have other types of migrainous episodes.

BAM produces a wide constellation of focal symptoms and signs all of which are referrable to the posterior cerebral hemispheres, cerebellum and brainstem. Bickerstaff (1986) has, however, expressed concern that the extension and expansion of the range of original symptoms described (Bickerstaff, 1961a) has led to situations in which the diagnosis of BAM is a 'singularly tenuous one'. As the involvement of the posterior circulation is common in many forms of migrainous attacks, Lapkin and Golden (1978) have suggested the division of patients into three groups. Their third group is defined as 'episodic headache and/or a strong family history of migraine and three or more recurrent neurological symptoms referrable to the basilar–vertebral arterial tree'. It is this third group that conforms to what is generally accepted as BAM. An early age of onset is now well described in children with BAM, together with a very high incidence of positive family histories. The differential diagnosis for BAM is wide and in the absence of a positive family history or a history of similar attacks, structural abnormalities of the posterior fossa and a wide range of metabolic disorders have to be considered. The outlook for most children with BAM is good, although many will at a later age go on to develop more classical migrainous attacks. Hockaday (1979) has, however, pointed out that in those with a particularly early onset of attacks, the outlook for neurological development may not always be favourable.

Ophthalmoplegic migraine may occur at a very young age and must always raise the question of the existence of an aneurysm. Existing data does, however, point very clearly to the extreme rarity of such a possibility. Differentiation from the presumed granulomatous disorder of Tolosa–Hunt may be difficult and, therefore, some have argued that treatment with steroids should always be considered, particularly as in some children it is well documented that recovery may be incomplete.

Elements of confusion, altered consciousness and behaviour occur in many differing forms of migrainous episodes. However, in so-called confusional migraine these elements are the most prominent, with other migrainous symptoms such as headache being less apparent, particularly at the time the child presents. It is perhaps with confusional migraine that the greatest care is needed in excluding an alternative diagnosis. Barlow (1984) has emphasized that drug ingestion is far more likely to be an explanation for an acute confusional episode in children than is migraine. Nevertheless, other metabolic, inflammatory, epileptic and psychogenic causes must additionally be actively considered.

In most reviews of complicated migraine of childhood mention is rightly made of difficulty in eliciting a history of headache. In some this may not be a prominent symptom and with individual attacks it may be absent. In the very young child the specific symptoms that characterize a particular form of migraine may be difficult to elucidate because of the age of the child. This inevitably produces underdiagnosis of complicated migraine but at the same time it leads to an urgent search for alternative diagnoses. However, within all this it is important that the clinician does appreciate that complicated migraines do occur even in very young children and infants, so that investigations, particularly invasive ones, are used judiciously rather than always exhaustively.

Chapter 4

Equivalents of childhood migraine

Judith M. Hockaday

We construct such boundaries and limits for there is none in the subject itself. (Sacks, 1970)

Introduction

It is important to distinguish between so-called equivalents of migraine and variants of migraine. A *variant* of migraine is an unusual form which however fulfills usual diagnostic criteria in a migraine subject (see Chapter 3). An *equivalent* is 'an episodic transient dysfunction in a migraine patient which is not closely tied to the migraine attack, indeed may completely replace the attack' (Bruyn, 1986): an equivalent of migraine is essentially migraine without headache.

In some discussions no specific meanings have been intended for the terms variant or equivalent. The phrases have been applied to a variety of recurrent and more or less stereotyped phenomena, of unknown cause, proposed as forms of, or associations with, migraine, and are used particularly in relation to childhood disorders such as the periodic syndrome, cyclical vomiting, recurrent abdominal pain, bilious attacks and 'abdominal migraine'. These are all ill-defined disorders and the descriptions and distinctions made by different authors are therefore arbitrary, and sometimes unclear. A comparative review of the literature is correspondingly difficult.

There are other paroxysmal phenomena of early childhood which may be related to migraine, as associations, or as alternative or early expressions of it: for example, some recurrent paroxysmal torticollis syndromes, some benign paroxysmal vertiginous syndromes and the alternating hemiplegia syndrome. These disorders are rare but important. The evidence linking any one of them with migraine is slight, but the disorders are more clearly defined than the syndromes referred to above, and they are therefore discussed separately in Chapter 6. Other disorders sometimes considered to occur as associations of migraine, such as travel sickness and somnambulism, are referred to in Chapter 1.

Migraine without headache

Migraine is a disorder in which headache is by ordinary definition the essential feature. However, headache is only one symptom of many and neurological abnormalities are common: these include mental, motor, sensory and autonomic disturbances. The importance of headache in diagnosis is recognized in all definitions (for example, Vahlquist, 1955; Friedman *et al.*, 1962a; World Federation of Neurology, 1969). Nevertheless, attacks of migraine without headache although probably uncommon are well recognized and well described in the literature (Selby and Lance, 1960; Whitty, 1967; Bruyn, 1986). Thus Whitty (1967) reported 16 cases collected from a very large series of migraine over many years: he included three with symptoms from a young age (14 years) consisting of fortification spectra, visual blurring with dysphasia, and numbness, weakness and tingling of the left arm, face and tongue, all without ensuing headache. In his survey of childhood migraine Bille (1962) accepted that migraine without headache might occur: 'aura symptoms might occur as an equivalent for many years without the child having any typical migraine attacks,' and he recorded 'scintillations without scotoma,' without subsequent headache, in 11% of 73 children with severe migraine.

Any neurological dysfunction occurring in the aura of migraine may occur in isolation, without ensuing headache – other names for this phenomenon are abortive migraine and migraine dissociée. The most frequent is recurrent scintillating scotomata but other visual distortions, and sensory and motor and mental symptoms are also described (reviewed by Bruyn, 1986). The clinical diagnosis of these episodes of neurological dysfunction without headache as migraine equivalents is, of course, acceptable only after full investigation, and when detailed enquiry and follow-up reveals typical migraine (with headache) in the past or future course: even then the identity of the so-called equivalent with migraine cannot be proven.

The problem is even more difficult when considering other symptoms known to occur before or during migraine attacks. Some of the autonomic disturbances and so-called vegetative visceral symptoms are by their nature more ill defined than the neurological symptoms typical of the aura. The proposal that they also can occur in isolation without ensuing or accompanying headache is reasonable and many accept that this occurs. This may or may not be so. As there is no diagnostic test for common migraine, and only (recently) a not readily available 'test' for classical migraine (Olesen, 1986), and as even the common identity of these two conditions is not established (Wilkinson, 1986), the chances of reaching a conclusion on so-called visceral equivalents of migraine seem remote at the present time. However, a considerable body of well-informed opinion accepts their reality (Barlow, 1984; Bruyn, 1986), and many recurrent syndromes of childhood are currently treated with antimigraine remedies. The uncertainties of diagnosis are such that very careful attention needs to be given to other diagnostic possibilities first.

Prevalence

It is difficult to obtain a measure of the prevalence of equivalents of migraine in childhood. In the author's experience specific neurological symptoms/equivalents such as attacks of teichopsia or metamorphopsia without ensuing headache are rare in children considered on other grounds to have migraine, and so is a history of attacks of gastrointestinal disturbance without headache – so-called abdominal migraine. When due account is taken of the difficulties sometimes experienced by small children in identifying or localizing pain, especially to the head, many apparent examples of equivalents of migraine will prove to be acceptable as ordinary migraine. Young children may not have learnt to localize pain, and they may neither have the vocabulary to describe a sensation as painful nor be able to characterize pain by its location, for example as tummyache, headache or earache. Often careful interpretation of a child's behaviour and gesture may indicate that headache is indeed part of a symptom complex at first thought to be gastrointestinal only. Again in older children whose symptoms are dominated by prostration and vomiting specific enquiry will often be necessary before an account of headache is obtained. Complete absence of headache in attacks considered on other grounds to be migraine is probably quite uncommon.

Visceral/vegetative symptoms during migraine attacks

When gastrointestinal symptoms occur with headache in a subject whose attack pattern is typical of migraine and who is otherwise well, there is little difficulty in accepting them as part of the migraine attack. They occur very commonly and, as the term 'sick headache' implies, nausea with or without vomiting is a useful diagnostic criterion. It was observed in 72 of 122 children by Hockaday (1979) and in 296 of 300 children by Congdon and Forsythe (1979). Vomiting without associated nausea is in contrast extremely uncommon, but was observed in four of 300 cases by Congdon and Forsythe (1979).

Anorexia, flatulence, hiccups, abdominal distension, constipation and diarrhoea are also all well known as accompaniments to a headache attack. Abdominal pain is less often described. Klee (1968) does not mention it in his very detailed clinical study and nor do Lance and Anthony (1966) in their survey of 500 patients. Herberg (1975) also does not mention abdominal pain in his lengthy review of hypothalamic function and 'vegetative symptoms', nor is it included by Blau (1980, 1986) in his exhaustive studies of complete migraine. H. Isler (1985, personal communication) has not observed abdominal pain as a premonitory symptom. However, Amery *et al.* (1986) listed abdominal pain among the prodromal symptoms of spontaneous attacks in four of 15 adults. Sacks (1970) observed that one in ten adults with common migraine may experience abdominal pain or abnormal bowel action during the course of an attack and that 'the proportion is notably higher in younger patients'. It may be that more detailed enquiry will elicit the complaint more frequently. Bille (1962) observed abdominal pain during the headache phase in 10% of children with what he called pronounced migraine (PMi). Prensky and Sommer (1979) also observed that abdominal pain was a very common complaint (19% of a hospital clinic childhood series): although the significance of this is modified by their use of the symptom as one of six criteria diagnostic of childhood migraine. Hockaday (1979) observed abdominal pain during the attack in five of 29 children with BAM and Congdon and Forsythe (1979) recorded it as part of the aura stage in 10% of children with classical migraine (4% of their series overall). Holquin and Fenichel (1967) had similar findings. Thus the observation of Sacks (1970) that abdominal pain may be a feature of the attack more commonly in younger subjects appears correct. Unfortunately in some of the papers cited there is little information about the nature of the pain and its position and duration, and timing is not always given in relation to the different parts of the migraine attack, thus it is not clear whether it is sometimes prodromal, part of the aura, or an association with the headache.

Abdominal migraine

There have been many reports of a high childhood incidence of abdominal pain, bilious attacks, cyclical vomiting, recurrent vomiting, periodic syndrome in migraine subjects studied retrospectively. These phenomena are sometimes all included within the term 'abdominal migraine' currently in common use. The study by Lance and Anthony (1966) is typical: they observed that 23% of adult migraineurs attending a headache clinic gave a past history of frequent vomiting attacks in childhood compared with only 12% of patients with tension headache. Lundberg (1975) found 12% of adult migraineurs had recurrent abdominal pain. However, in this ill-defined field, retrospective enquiry even in well-studied and well-controlled groups introduces unacceptable bias. There is unfortunately very little controlled prospectively collected information about abdominal or gastrointestinal equivalents of migraine. The most notable study in childhood is that of Bille (1962), who reported that 38% of children with severe migraine had equivalents defined as follows: 'in patients who have or have had migraine, the migraine attacks with headache may alternate with, or for a short or long period be replaced by, other paroxysmal disturbances of different kinds'. The most common equivalent was attacks of abdominal pains, recorded in 15 of the 73 children. Bille defined the attacks as being severe enough to affect activities and occurring at least three times over 'a fairly long period'. The nature, site and duration of the pain is not described. Apparently similar attacks were reported by only three of 73 non-migraine control children. Bille also included cyclical vomiting (undefined) as an equivalent, observed in three (boys) of 73 of his childhood migraine cases and not occurring in the control group.

It is difficult to obtain an estimate of the frequency of abdominal migraine. Sacks (1970) describes isolated cases. Symon and Russell (1986) do not describe the population from which they drew their large number of reported cases. In Bille's study (1962) the high incidence (20.5%) of abdominal pain syndrome was measured only in a group of 73 children selected by virtue of having severe migraine from 347 children with migraine in a school population of 9059 children aged 7–15 years. The incidence of equivalents in the whole migraine group, or in the other subgroups of this population, is not stated. In contrast to this, Congdon and Forsythe (1979) reported that only 10 of their 300 children with migraine of all types had experienced recurrent attacks of abdominal pain, without headache, before they started to have migraine.

It is possible that the incidence of prior or coincident 'unexplained' recurrent attacks of abdominal pain or other gastrointestinal upset in some headache groups is at the level expected in any childhood population. Indeed, Koch and Melchior (1969) observed more concomitant disorders such as abdominal pain and constipation ('of possible psychosomatic origin') in children with non-migraine headache than in those with migraine. Deubner (1977) studied 780 children aged 10–20 years, and found no excess of cyclic vomiting prior to age 10 reported by migraine subjects (one in 78) compared with headache-free subjects (seven in 87), nor of 'nervous vomiting', (seven in 72, compared with five in 89), nor of recurrent attacks of abdominal pain (nine in 70, compared with 11 in 83). They did note, however, that parents recalled recurrent abdominal pain prior to age 10 more often in the migraine group (16 of 36) than in the headache-free group (six of 116). An implication that parents' reports are more accurate is not borne out by other findings, for significantly more subjects than parents described specific features such as unilaterality and focal neurological symptoms ($P \leqslant 0.001$). Again, while Small and Waters (1974) found that teenage boys and girls with migraine had suffered from abdominal pain more often than headache-free subjects, in another study Moss and Waters (1974) did not find any significant difference. And neither of these reports observed any excess of a past history of bilious attacks in the migraine groups. Moreover when they looked at the accuracy of their enquiries by a retrospective questionnaire, they found very poor reproducibility on a question about prior abdominal pain attacks after a 2-month interval: only 32 of 58 teenage girls gave the same answer on both occasions. The observations of the National Childhood Development Study (Kurtz et al., 1984) on the natural history of headaches, migraine, and some migraine equivalents were prospective and therefore important. Its cohort of children born in 1958 has been studied at age 7, 11, 16 and 23 years. When the children were 16, their parents were interrogated by questionnaire about the occurrence of migraine and recurrent sick headaches in the previous 12 months. The authors reported that their findings 'lend support to the idea that migraine and "recurrent syndrome" are essentially the same condition'. The tabulated results of Kurtz et al. (1984) show vomiting or abdominal pain with or without headache recorded much more often in the past of young people experiencing sick headache at age 16 than in those experiencing headache without sickness. However, sick headache was defined as headache with anorexia, nausea or vomiting, and only 27% of the group with sick headache were considered to have migraine (on the chosen criteria of vomiting or specific visual disturbance). Moreover the sick headache group as a whole was found to experience significantly more problems of many sorts, including emotional disturbance and maladjustment, and were more likely to come from a low social class and deprived home backgrounds. This is not a feature in migraine (Waters, 1971; Deubner, 1977) and perhaps distinguishes the cases. Unfortunately the figures from the National Childhood Development Study were not analysed separately for those considered to have migraine.

At the other extreme, Salmon (1983) has described a very close relationship between early childhood recurrent abdominal syndromes without headache, and later migraine. He describes the pain of abdominal migraine as central: 'recurrent central (T10) abdominal pain, possibly cyclical and lasting 30 minutes to several days – a dull aching pain'. This description is based on his retrospective analysis of the symptoms recorded in the records of 176 children who had earlier (1960–1969) presented with diagnoses of periodic syndrome, cyclical vomiting, recurrent headaches, growing pains and bilious attacks. His view that the abdominal pain attacks were equivalents of migraine was based on his findings that 37 of the 51 who were successfully traced as adults then had classical migraine. However, allowing for bias in reply, this could just reflect normal adult prevalence and cannot be interpreted as evidence for his later statement (Salmon, 1985) that 'a definite relationship between abdominal migraine, cranial migraine and cyclical vomiting is demonstrated'. Nor can it be accepted without further study that *inter alia* periodic syndrome, cyclical vomiting, grumbling appendix, growing pains, bilious attacks are 'now known to be synonymous with migraine'. Further, the use by Salmon (1983) and many others of a positive history of migraine in a family member as a diagnostic feature of abdominal migraine is not acceptable in clinical practice because of the very high background prevalence of migraine in the population.

It is thus difficult to prove from group studies that so-called abdominal migraine is a precursor to, or association with, migraine. However, there is a wealth of opinion that this is the case. The description and opinion of Sacks (1970) are authoritative and convincing; he states: 'the dominant feature of abdominal migraine is epigastric pain of continuous character and great severity', and he refers to cases where the pain lasted for many hours, even up to 10 h in one instance. Symon and Russell (1986) described 40 children with abdominal migraine in some detail. Unfortunately the size of the population from which these cases were drawn is not given. They describe the pain as mid-line, lasting for at least 2 h, of sufficient severity to stop normal activities and accompanied by vasomotor symptoms or nausea. Elsewhere in the paper attack duration is described as 6 h or longer. All their cases had a family history of migraine in first or second degree relatives (however this was a criterion for selection). Anorexia, nausea and vomiting were common. Nearly half also had migraine headaches: it is not stated whether these were coincident. Further study and follow-up of these cases will provide useful information. However, the view of Symon and Russell (1986) that 'the modification of the natural history of the disease in those patients treated with pizotifen is additional circumstantial evidence that the syndrome is related to migraine' is not acceptable in an area notoriously susceptible to placebo effect (*Lancet,* 1982). The same criticism should be held against this implication in a report of the benefits of pizotifen in five selected cases of cyclical vomiting reported by Salmon and Walters (1985).

Follow-up studies

In follow-up studies, a psychosomatic basis for most otherwise unexplained recurrent abdominal pain syndromes is generally accepted, and is well discussed by Berger *et al.* (1977), Nicol (1982), Coulthard (1984) and O'Donnell (1985). A recent study (McGrath *et al.,* 1983) failed to show any statistically significant differences between a group of children with RAP and a group of pain-free children, all referred to a gastroenterology clinic and analysed for stress factors, history of family pain and problems of personality. However, as the authors point out, there were consistent trends to more depression and immaturity in the children with pain, and, most importantly, children with factors clearly suggesting a psychogenic origin for the pain would not have been referred to the clinic. The role of stressful life events is discussed by Monaghon and Dodge (1980). In most studies, migraine is not a prominent sequel. The study by Salmon 1983 (see above) is a notable exception and so is that of Hammond (1974): she reviewed 12 adults who had been admitted to hospital in early life with a diagnosis of (unexplained) cyclical vomiting, and observed that eight developed migraine in adult life. Others have not observed this sequence. Reinhart *et al.* (1977) followed 16 subjects with childhood cyclical vomiting into early adult life and observed that all had psychosomatic problems but none had headache. Apley and Hale (1973) observed only three of 60 RAP subjects later developed migraine. Stickler and Murphy (1979) included headache as one form of 'hypochondriacal adjustment' in less than 17% of a large series. Christensen and Mortensen (1975) noted that headache, often migrainous, was a feature in some of their series at follow-up, together with a variety of symptoms such as back pain and bad nerves. An interesting finding in their paper was that offspring of subjects who were still symptomatic had a high incidence of RAP while offspring of those who had become symptom free were themselves symptom free. A recent long-term follow-up study for 10 or more years of 16 of 22 adults who had been admitted to hospital in early childhood for RAP found that 50% continued to have RAP or developed other painful symptoms, this poor outcome relating to identifiable social and personality features including living in 'painful families' (Magni *et al.*, 1987). Only one of the 16 later developed migraine. *Against this background, an opinion on whether unexplained RAP syndromes are 'migraine without headache' would be arbitrary and valueless.*

Problems

The question might seem at first glance of theoretical interest only. However, it is a matter of clinical importance. Syndromes regarded as visceral equivalents of migraine include many commonly occurring childhood disorders. On the assumption that they represent migraine, specific antimigraine remedies are frequently prescribed for them – ergotamine preparations, pizotifen and phenytoin are often recommended. Some authors recommend the use of these drugs as a 'therapeutic trial to confirm the diagnosis'. None has been shown by controlled trial to be of value for any of these ill-defined disorders and all carry the risk of undesirable side-effects (Wilkinson, 1984).

Differential diagnosis

There are other even more important clinical reasons for exercising caution in allowing the concept of abdominal migraine or regarding this form of periodic syndrome as an equivalent of migraine. As long ago as 1967 Mitchell wrote: 'the aetiological homogeneity of periodic disease becomes increasingly suspect as more and more features are identified and excluded'. This is still the case today, and syndromes identified as the periodic syndrome and abdominal migraine are still what is left over after ascertainable causes for the symptoms have been excluded. Diagnosis is therefore still arbitrary, depending on the accuracy and extent of investigation, and changing as knowledge advances.

A recent study (Tal *et al.*, 1984) considered that the diagnosis of abdominal migraine should be regarded with some reserve, citing two children thought to have abdominal migraine who were later found to have, respectively, *coeliac disease* and a *urea cycle disorder* (Rowe *et al.*, 1986). The differential diagnosis of syndromes with recurring abdominal pain and vomiting also includes disorders requiring extensive neurological investigation. In the author's recent experience, a child referred for further advice about medication for repeated abdominal pain labelled as 'abdominal migraine' proved to have *temporal lobe epilepsy,* successfully treated by temporal lobectomy, and another boy previously treated as having psychogenic (cyclical) vomiting was found on investigation to have a temporal lobe glioma (case detail kindly supplied by Dr Oxbury). A girl diagnosed for many years as having 'bilious attacks, periodic syndrome' proved to have a *mitochondrial cytopathy,* and a boy who had been under psychiatric care for 4 years because of periodic anorexia, vomiting and upper (hepatic) abdominal pain was also found to have a mitochondrial lesion (with hepatic pain associated with severe lactic acidosis). All these children had been attending hospital paediatric departments, and they illustrate the dangers and *uncertainties* of the notion that the various syndromes included under the label of periodic syndrome have any diagnostic validity. There is always a risk that applying a specific term such as abdominal migraine, periodic syndrome, or cyclical vomiting, prematurely, will prevent adequate investigation and identification of conditions such as the above, and of course of commoner disorders such as urinary tract infection.

In particular, the possibility that periodic abdominal symptoms are *epileptic* in origin should always be considered. Millichap *et al.* drew attention to 'cyclic vomiting as a form of epilepsy' as early as 1955. Abdominal and rising sensations are common in epilepsy. Pain is rare however. In a study of the abdominal aura in 100 epileptic patients, Van Buren (1963) found the sensation described as painful in only eight. It was most often indescribable (20) but was compared to fear, nervousness or guilt in 16, nausea in 14, or tenseness, movement, pressure, emptiness, warmth, or other feelings in the remainder. The duration is not described; only 46 experienced migration of the abdominal sensation, virtually always upward. Young and Blume (1983) also found abdominal pain rare as an epileptic aura: only three of 858 epileptic subjects described abdominal pain, which was epigastric, at or just to the left of the mid-line and unlike other epileptic abdominal sensations, did not rise, but remained in the epigastrum until consciousness was lost. Clinical and EEG evidence characterized the epilepsy to be of temporal lobe origin. The term 'abdominal epilepsy' has been used for a syndrome in which paroxysmal abdominal pain is associated with altered awareness, EEG abnormality and response to antiepileptic medication (Douglas and White, 1971). The concept is probably unnecessary (O'Donohoe, 1971) and abdominal sensations should only be considered epileptic when the diagnosis of epilepsy stands on other grounds including alteration of awareness or responsiveness. Douglas and White (1971) considered the abdominal pain of so-called abdominal epilepsy to be of relatively short duration – a few minutes, compared with the more prolonged abdominal symptoms described in migraine (Sacks, 1970). The distinction can be difficult, however, particularly in young children. Some children with very frequent complex partial seizures ('status') may complain at length and repeatedly only of ill-defined tummyaches: their periods of altered consciousness, with or without automatisms, may be misinterpreted as the behaviour of a distressed child.

Conclusion

The majority of physicians experienced in childhood migraine recognize (rare) cases where, over a period of some years, attacks of unexplained abdominal pain prolonged for up to many hours and associated with pallor, lethargy, nausea and perhaps vomiting, are replaced gradually or suddenly, by attacks with headache. At this point a retrospective clinical diagnosis of 'abdominal migraine' may be considered. Before this point so-called abdominal migraine cannot be identified.

Despite the large literature, and widely held opinion that some of the paroxysmal gastrointestinal disorders of childhood are 'equivalents' of migraine, it would be unwise to accept that 'abdominal migraine' can be a well-based clinical diagnosis at the present time.

Summary

All definitions of migraine include headache as an essential part of the symptom complex, and recognize that extracranial symptoms (visceral/vegetative) are common, and that a neurological aura may occur. It is also well recognized that occasionally the headache part of the symptom complex may be absent: the episode is then regarded as a migraine equivalent (migraine without headache). When in this situation an attack consists of neurological symptoms characteristic of migraine, for example scintillating scotoma, in a subject known to have had migraine in the past, or established as having migraine at later review, then the attack may be regarded with some justification as an equivalent of migraine. However, when an attack consists of less well defined neurological or visceral/vegetative symptoms, there must always be considerable doubt about its nature, unless or until the same symptoms later recur as part of typical migraine.

The alternative diagnoses for one or more episodes of neurological disturbance are clearly important, for example epilepsy, and cerebral tumour. The alternative diagnoses for recurrent visceral symptoms are no less important, including for example intussusception, urea cycle disorders, mitochondrial cytopathies, and complex partial seizures. There are no specific features which distinguish the extracranial symptoms of migraine. They should be regarded as equivalents of migraine only when the diagnosis of migraine is clear on other grounds *and* when full investigation has excluded other causes. Use of the term abdominal migraine for recurring symptom complexes which may or may not be migraine is unhelpful, implying more certainty than can at present exist.

Chapter 5

Management of childhood migraine

Ian Forsythe and Judith M. Hockaday

Introduction

Migraine is more common in children than most doctors realize, occurring in 2–4.5% (Sillanpåå, 1976). The attacks may be frequent and severe in 40% and especially severe in children who are awakened at night with their attacks: 4% of cases in one series (Congdon and Forsythe, 1979). Therefore, it is important that neurologists, paediatricians and medical practitioners, if they are to be successful in the treatment of childhood migraine, show a genuine interest in the patient's distress by allowing the parent and patient sufficient time to discuss symptoms and the effects they have on school work and in the home. The importance of trigger factors can be considered as well as the patient's psychological state and ability to relax.

It is always important to discover the reason for the consultation. Many parents associate recurrent headaches with head trauma or with brain tumour, and their reason for consultation may well be anxiety about this possibility, rather than concern about the severity of the child's symptoms. Some 17% of children with migraine present with early morning headache and vomiting (Congdon and Forsythe, 1979). A detailed history, clinical (including neurological) examination, with measurement of blood pressure and examination of the fundi, is always necessary. A CT scan should be obtained if a space-occupying lesion is suspected. Indications for investigation are discussed in Chapter 1. In many cases reassurance that the headaches are not due to a brain tumour may enable the parents to cope with the child's migraine with minimal medical help.

Many active and prophylactic treatments have been recommended for childhood and adult migraine but the fact that there are so many attests to its generally unsatisfactory management. No agent is effective in all patients and several patients prove refractory to all remedies. When reporting results of treatment it is essential that migraine is defined. Classical migraine usually presents no difficulty, but it is important to remember that many children with classical migraine have in addition, and sometimes more frequently, attacks of common migraine. Several weeks of accurate recording of attacks may be necessary before BAM can be diagnosed, and its differentiation from epilepsy confirmed. Tension headaches occur in childhood and it may be impossible to differentiate an attack of common migraine from a tension headache; a unilateral headache does not exclude the latter diagnosis, and, often, both occur in the same child.

Unlike adult migraineurs, between 30% and 40% of children with migraine grow out of their complaint (Bille, 1962; Prensky, 1976; Congdon and Forsythe, 1979).

Attacks can stop suddenly or slowly diminish in frequency and severity, and with such a high spontaneous remission rate it is essential that double-blind trials are undertaken to evaluate treatment.

Avoiding attacks

Trigger factors

There appears to be no doubt that, on a basis of constitutional predisposition, certain trigger mechanisms appear to precipitate attacks of migraine (or tension headache). The following factors, many stress related, may be relevant: anxiety, examinations, family tension, late nights, minor head trauma, fasting, dietary constituents, sex hormone variations, bright light, sunlight, television, disco-theques, loud noise, cold weather, and there are many others (Vahlquist, 1955; Bille, 1962; Congdon and Forsythe, 1979; Maratos and Wilkinson, 1982). Vahlquist (1955) and Maratos and Wilkinson (1982) reported that as many as 80% and 86% of attacks, respectively, were precipitated by emotional upset. Bille (1962) found that 31% of his patients were able to identify school work, especially examinations, as a factor in their headaches. It has been suggested that 'dyslexia' and other learning problems are important trigger factors, especially in boys, but more research is needed before the importance of learning problems in childhood migraine can be evaluated.

Many of the so-called trigger factors are not very specific, and they can be inconsistent, so that although they are effective on some occasions, they are harmless on others. They may therefore be difficult to identify. Parents may well be unaware of trigger factors, and children often have difficulty in recognizing or describing them. Because of this a school report, if possible from a teacher personally involved with the child, should be obtained as a matter of routine: accounts of unexpected teasing and bullying, and learning difficulties, often emerge. Stress factors outside school may not be immediately obvious, and this is particularly the case when a child experiences family strife, or is the subject of abuse, verbal or physical, or deprivation within the family.

Bille (1962) advised that maintaining sound biological rhythms in terms of life, work, rest, meals and sleep should be followed. However, if careful records are kept before and after removal of trigger factors, results are frequently disappointing. Similarly, when a patient obtains full remission the so-called trigger factors which were originally identified are generally still present in most cases. Trigger factors are discussed more fully in Chapter 8.

Diet factors

In 1925 it was reported that migraine could be precipitated by certain foodstuffs: alcohol, cheese, chocolate, coffee, eggs, fish, fruit, game, meat extracts, milk, mushrooms, poultry, sweetbreads, tea and tomatoes (Curtis-Brown, 1925). Interest was reawakened when it was suggested that tyramine-containing foodstuffs could precipitate an attack of migraine (Hanington, 1967). Tyramine, a naturally occurring substance, is known to release serotonin from platelets. However, doubt about the relevance of foodstuffs containing tyramine to migraine was raised by negative double-blind studies of tyramine and placebo in children (Forsythe and Redmond, 1974; Congdon and Forsythe, 1979), and in adults (Ryan, 1974; Ziegler and Stewart, 1977; see Chapter 8 for further discussion). In the childhood studies, Congdon and Forsythe (1979) reported that of 80 children, 22 had a headache after receiving tyramine, whereas 34 developed a headache after receiving placebo. Another suggestion was that phenylethylamine was the responsible agent in chocolate (which contains very little tyramine), because patients with chocolate-induced migraine were found to have headaches after administration of phenylethylamine (Sandler et al., 1974). Phenylethylamine and tyramine are vasoactive amines and may act directly on the cranial vasculature or they may cause release of 5-hydroxytryptamine (5-HT) from platelets or alter noradrenaline metabolism. Two subsequent studies showed that the concentration of phenylethylamine in chocolate was much lower than originally reported and the significance of phenylethylamine as a headache-provoking factor remains in doubt (Schweitzer et al., 1975; Hurst and Toomey, 1981). A reduction of platelet phenol sulphotransferase activity has been demonstrated in patients with dietary migraine (Littlewood et al., 1982). It is suggested that foods associated with migraine contain an unidentified phenolic substrate of the enzyme. The importance of vasoactive amines in the precipitation of attacks of migraine in children remains in considerable doubt. A recent study (Salfield et al., 1987) found no significant difference between the effects of a vasoactive amine-free, and a control, high-fibre diet.

In 1983 it was claimed that 93% of 88 children with severe and frequent migraine recovered on an oligoantigenic diet (Egger et al., 1983). Over 50 foods were identified: cows milk in 27, eggs in 24, wheat and oranges each in 21, and tomatoes and cheese each in 13 patients. In several patients multiple foods were responsible. In a similar study of 52 children with frequent and severe migraine treated with an elimination diet for 3 weeks, followed by careful food reintroduction in those children who showed a marked reduction in frequency and severity of their attacks while on the diet (Macdonald et al., 1987), the diagnosis of food intolerance was considered proven if a positive reaction to two open and one blind challenge was obtained. Only seven (13%) were considered on these grounds to have food intolerance. Eight (15%) had a 'spontaneous remission' as soon as they were shown the diet sheet, and six of these remained in remission for more than a year. All eight had a history of one or more attacks of migraine per week for 1–6 years. Many unexpected problems were encountered. It was essential that an expert dietitian kept in close contact with the mother, at least once a week, otherwise mistakes were common. It was difficult for older children to maintain their nutritional needs on such a limited diet. An elimination diet costs two to three times more than a normal diet (MacDonald and Forsythe, 1986) and because of this high cost it has been modified to exclude only milk, eggs, some additives and vasoactive amine-containing foods; only if the symptoms persist, and the child and parents are motivated, is the stricter elimination diet tried. Undoubtedly, the elimination diet is the best diagnostic tool when dealing with multiple food intolerance but the problems accompanying it are numerous, and it is important to consider all factors before recommending its use in children.

Over and beyond these clinical implications of the use of diagnostic elimination diets are the problems of methodology and interpretation which at present are generally not adequately allowed for (Leviton, 1984; Pearson, 1985; see Chapter 8). When careful methodology is observed, then findings are often negative, as was recently shown, for example, in a study of the effect of dietary tartrazine on behaviour (David, 1987).

Treatment

Although there is no complete and satisfactory cure for migraine, apart from a spontaneous remission, much can be done to help almost every patient. The type of therapy will depend on the severity and frequency of attacks and in children these may vary widely. If the attacks are infrequent, and not severe, all that is required is reassurance and an analgesic. However, if the attacks are severe and recur more than twice per month prophylactic treatment should be considered. Each case must be considered individually however. Occasionally even infrequent attacks warrant prophylactic therapy, for example, to protect the child at important times such as when taking examinations. Again, if attacks are prolonged and distressing, or associated with prominent neurological features, or there is held to be a risk of residual permanent abnormality, then preventive treatment should be considered.

In general, parents should be advised to see what benefits follow clear diagnosis and reassurance, and symptomatic treatment of attacks as they arise, before embarking on preventive medication. Many are so reassured by finding simple measures effective that no further treatment is necessary. Many are sufficiently reassured by knowing the natural high remission rate for children. Many parents recognize that the main disability, and the real reason for medical consultation, is the anxiety the attacks cause – once this is relieved, they see no need for preventive medication. Many recognize that occasional headaches constitute a lesser problem than regular medication and all can benefit from understanding that there is a wide range of medicaments which can be tried if necessary.

Before starting treatment it is important to clarify the relationships between the child's disability from attacks of migraine, and schooling. Difficulties in personal relationships or in academic progress are common in all school communities, and an account of school problems often emerges in children with migraine. The link with school failure may not be direct: Collin et al. (1985) found less than 1% of school absence overall was due to headache, and that duration of absence due to headache very rarely exceeded a single day (see Chapter 1). When migraine and school failure appear to be linked often the primary problem is a learning difficulty, with migraine provoked or exacerbated by the difficulty and offered as a more acceptable reason for presentation. The distinction between frequent common migraine occurring in this situation and tension headache may be difficult, or indeed not possible; often both occur. The relationships between migraine and schooling are however complex. It is important to recognize the children in whom frequent severe headaches are symptomatic of school refusal, or other psychiatric disorder: repeated recall for special investigation and repeated trials of different medicaments are contraindicated in such disorders.

Treatment of the acute attack

Treatment should be given as soon as possible after the start of the attack. Parents should be encouraged to learn to suspect when an attack is imminent by observing prodromal changes in, for example, mood, behaviour, appetite, or sleep pattern, so that treatment may be started at this stage. Prodromal symptoms, that is, symptoms other than those of a focal neurological aura, preceding the headache stage sometimes by many hours, were reported by Klee (1968) in 14%, and by Blau (1980) in 20% of cases (see Chapter 1).

It is customary to advise rest, and analgesic treatment (aspirin or paracetamol) in readily soluble form, together with an antiemetic preparation (e.g. metoclopramide) given beforehand, parenterally if necessary. In the authors' experience, rest in a darkened room and analgesic therapy, are generally sufficient, and metoclopramide is of doubtful additional value in children. There is no place for the use of strong analgesic drugs. Calorie and fluid intake should be maintained if possible. In children of school age, if attacks arise during the school day, a darkened room should be available, and analgesic medication should be allowed at once, so that the child may recover rapidly, and return to class after only a short break, so avoiding being sent home. Congdon and Forsythe (1979) found that 39% of children have one or more attacks per week: for these, provision of adequate facilities in school is essential.

Medication
Analgesics will relieve the majority of migraine headaches, if taken early, and if absorbed. Recommended preparations include paracetamol, in tablet or liquid preparation, and aspirin as dispersible or effervescent tablets; occasionally codeine phosphate may be used, again in tablet or syrup form. The use of aspirin for children aged 12 years and under with migraine is precluded, because of uncertainty about its role in the aetiology of Reye's syndrome (except in rare special circumstances, e.g. in attempts at control of some severe complicated forms of migraine).

It has long been recognized that gastric stasis and prolongation of gastric emptying occurs during a migraine attack (Carstairs, 1958). Some analgesics have been combined with antiemetics, for example, paracetamol and codeine with buclizine hydrochloride, and paracetamol or aspirin with metoclopramide. It has been shown that metoclopramide facilitates gastric emptying and absorption of paracetamol (Nimmo *et al.*, 1973) and of aspirin (Volans, 1975; Wainscott *et al.*, 1976), but any superior clinical benefit of combination preparations of analgesics with metoclopramide or other drugs remains unproven (*Drug and Therapeutics Bulletin*, 1980, 1981). However, in difficult cases it may be helpful to try different preparations in turn, until the most effective is found. It should be noted that in two children in the elimination diet study referred to above (MacDonald *et al.*, 1987) attacks of migraine were thought to have been precipitated by an aspirin-containing preparation.

At both the Princess Margaret Migraine Clinic in London (Wilkinson *et al.*, 1978) and the Copenhagen Acute Headache Clinic (Olesen *et al.*, 1979) an analgesic (aspirin or paracetamol) and diazepam (5 mg) are given by mouth to all patients on arrival, and all patients who are admitted are treated in addition with metoclopramide (10 mg) given by mouth or intramuscularly. The London Clinic claimed that diazepam (or other sedative) was helpful, because a higher percentage of patients receiving sedation were found to be improved. However, the Copenhagen group were more cautious and were unable to say whether their good results were due to the drugs or the clinic setting. In a later study from the Copenhagen Clinic Tfelt-Hansen *et al.* (1980) compared metoclopramide 10 mg i.m., metoclopramide 20 mg as suppository, and placebo, in a double-blind trial in patients also given paracetamol 1 g and diazepam 5 mg by mouth. Metoclopramide appeared to enhance the effect of the analgesic/sedative medication. Adverse affects of metoclopramide and similar drugs include important CNS reactions, and this appears to be a risk particularly in children, even in those given low doses.

Casteels-van Daele *et al.* (1970) and Gatrad (1976) described severe and unpleasant dystonic reactions including oculogyric crises in children. It should therefore be used with caution, and only after due warning to parents.

A small number of children with migraine (4% in the first author's own series; Congdon and Forsythe, 1979) are woken at night by severe headache; although vomiting may be followed by relief of symptoms and return to sleep, this does not always happen. Rectal diazepam, better absorbed than diazepam given orally, should be considered for this sort of case: indeed a double-blind controlled study is needed to assess the efficacy of diazepam given rectally at the onset of attacks in severe migraine in general.

Ergotamine   It is claimed that ergotamine tartrate is the most effective treatment to end an attack (Trued, 1974), although this has been questioned recently (Thrush, 1984). Numerous preparations are available (*Drug and Therapeutics Bulletin*, 1981), which may be administered orally, sublingually, rectally or by inhalation. Ergot is poorly absorbed from the gastrointestinal tract and a sublingual or effervescent preparation of ergotamine is often better. Dihydroergotamine has to be given in higher doses than ergotamine to end an attack, but its weaker vasoconstrictive action allows it to be used on a long-term basis. When caffeine is combined with ergot there appears to be better absorption of the latter. Side-effects of ergotamine preparations, including nausea, vomiting, muscle cramps and headache, can be unpleasant, and with prolonged use disabling (Wilkinson, 1984). In an effort to assess the effectiveness of ergotamine inhalers and tablets versus placebo inhalers and tablets 111 children were included in a double-blind crossover study (Congdon and Forsythe, 1979). The study lasted 7 years; unfortunately the drop-out rate of 66% precluded any statistical treatment of results. However, an objective analysis of the 38 children who completed all four treatment regimens did not suggest that any treatment was superior to another. A similar experience was obtained with 60 children treated with dihydroergotamine, and its use is no longer recommended for childhood migraine.

Other drugs   Other drugs, many with antiemetic action, have been tried. The phenothiazines chlorpromazine, 10–25 mg thrice daily by mouth, or 25 mg twice daily by suppository, and prochlorperazine maleate 10 mg daily by mouth are recommended but have not been tested by controlled trial. In addition to its use in treatment of the acute attack prochlorperazine is often used as a preventive drug: again its value is not proven. Another antiemetic, domperidone, has not been tested in children with migraine. Propranolol, also tried in acute attacks in adults (Tokola and Hokkanen, 1978), has not been studied in this way in children.

When more than 400 remedies have been used for the acute and prophylactic treatment of migraine in adults (Parkes, 1975) it is not surprising that sedatives and tranquillizers have been recommended. A sedative has a calming effect on the CNS, but does not induce sleep or analgesia. A review of the literature since 1963 has yielded considerable anecdotal evidence of the value of sedatives, but none has been evaluated in a double-blind trial in adults or children (Forsythe, 1986). Tranquillizers such as the benzodiazepine drugs relieve emotional stress, disturbed behaviour and symptoms causing clouding of consciousness (*Butterworths Medical Dictionary*, 1978). Although used in adult migraine it is fortunate that few paediatricians recommend their use in prophylaxis of childhood migraine because of the risk of addiction and withdrawal symptoms (Maletzky and Klotter, 1976).

Prophylactic treatment

No child should be subjected to continuous prophylactic medication unless the attacks of migraine are severe and frequent (more than two per month), or in special circumstances. Careful records must be kept of frequency, duration and severity of attacks, systemic upset and side-effects. Parents should be made aware of the more important side-effects.

There is a great variety of drugs reported as having preventive action in migraine, but responses of adults, and even more so of children, have been variable. The remedies most used in children are described here. For fuller information see Anthony (1983) and Peatfield (1986).

Propranolol
Propranolol is a beta-adrenergic blocking drug which among its other actions affects release of serotonin from platelets. Timolol, with similar actions, has also been used in children. Propranolol should be given in three divided doses daily, because the plasma half-life is short. Side-effects include rashes, insomnia, diarrhoea, increased appetite and weight gain. Known contraindications include a history or signs of obstructive airway disease, heart failure, cardiac conduction defect or other cardiac abnormality. There have been several controlled studies of the effect of propranolol in adults, with good results (Stensrud and Sjaastad, 1980; Weerasuriya *et al.*, 1982). Benefit may be due in part to an anxiolytic or anti-5HT action.

The value of propranolol or other beta blockers in children is not established. Ludvigsson (1974) reported that in a double-blind crossover trial in 28 children aged 7–16 years, comparing propranolol 60–120 mg daily and placebo, 20 children had a complete remission while on propranolol whereas only three had a complete remission while on placebo; insomnia was a problem in only two children. In contrast, in another double-blind controlled study of 39 children, Forsythe *et al.* (1984) found no significant difference between those treated with propranolol and those given placebo as regards frequency, severity or duration of attacks: indeed there was some evidence that propranolol increased the average duration of attacks. Again, in a double-blind controlled study comparing propranolol and placebo in 28 children with classical migraine, Olness *et al.* (1987) found the mean number of headaches per child for 3 months during the propranolol period was 14.9, compared with 13.3 during the placebo period. In a study of another beta blocker Noronha (1985) found no difference between the effects of timotol maleate and placebo in a controlled study in 17 children.

Clonidine
Clonidine affects central vasomotor reflexes and alters the reactivity of blood vessels to vasoconstrictor and vasodilator stimuli; it is therefore considered to modify the vascular changes occurring in a migraine attack. It is used in low dose in migraine, compared with its use in the treatment of hypertension. Administration should be in two or three divided doses daily. Unwanted effects include depression, dryness of the mouth, sedation and dizziness. It should not be used in pregnancy, nor in the presence of glaucoma or urinary retention. In a study in adults Ryan *et al.* (1975) found no significant differences in a double-blind controlled comparison of clonidine and placebo. The benefit of clonidine in children is also in doubt. In a pilot study in 50 children with migraine treated with clonidine for 2–15 months,

average 6 months, Sills *et al.* (1982) found that 20 obtained complete relief and remained in remission on average for 3 years. However, in a later double-blind study of an additional 43 children, there was no significant difference between those treated with clonidine or placebo as regards frequency, duration or severity of attacks, thus emphasizing the importance of the placebo effect and the necessity for double-blind studies in children (Sills *et al.*, 1982).

Pizotifen
Pizotifen has potent antiserotonin, antihistamine, and weak anticholinergic actions. It has an elimination half-life of 23 h, and may be given once daily. Side-effects include drowsiness, nausea, increased appetite and weight gain, which can cause considerable problems in children. Pizotifen should not be used in pregnancy or given to patients with glaucoma or urinary retention. There have been several double-blind studies demonstrating the effectiveness of pizotifen in adults. Experience of its use in children is limited however, and, at the present time, the place of pizotifen in treatment of childhood migraine is not established in controlled study. In one such study, of 39 children given pizotifen 0.5 mg twice or thrice daily, Gillies *et al.* (1986) found no significant difference between pizotifen and placebo treatments as regards frequency, duration and severity of attacks. In another study from the same centre 25 children with migraine were included in a double-blind study with pizotifen 1.5 mg or placebo given at night. None of the children had previous drug prophylaxis. Again there was no significant difference between pizotifen and placebo treatments as regards frequency, duration or severity of attacks (P. C. Ng *et al.*, 1987, personal communication).

In those children who obtained relief on active treatment in these two double-blind studies, active treatment was continued for 3–9 months (mean 7 months): 54% relapsed while on treatment or when it was withdrawn. A similar result was obtained with placebo remissions: 49% relapsed when treatment was withdrawn, again emphasizing the significant effect of placebo use in migraine.

Methysergide
Methysergide is an ergot derivative with potent serotonin receptor antagonism. It has been used widely as a prophylactic in adults (Fanchamps, 1975). However, it is not recommended for use in young children because of side-effects which include dizziness, muscle cramps, abnormal exudate and fibrosis, sometimes cardiac, or retroperitoneal causing impairment of renal function. In older children it may be used with caution (after other measures have proved unsuccessful), and it is important that treatment should be intermittent: continued for no longer than 4 months, with intervals of at least 1 month, to reduce the risks of fibrotic reactions. Contraindications to the use of methysergide include renal, vascular and cardiac disease.

Cyproheptadine
Cyproheptadine is better known as an antihistamine, but has serotonin blocking properties (Goodman and Gilman, 1970). Recent work has indicated that cyproheptadine also acts as a calcium-channel blocker (Peroutka and Allen, 1984). The recommended dosage is 30 mg twice daily. In a pilot study on 19 children, four had no attacks and 13 were much improved while on treatment (Bille *et al.*, 1977). Side-effects include drowsiness. Contraindications to its use are glaucoma, peptic ulcer and asthma. Unfortunately cyproheptadine has not been subjected to double-blind study in children.

Calcium-channel blockers
Yamamoto and Meyer (1980) suggested that calcium-channel blockers might relieve the aura and headache of classical migraine, because the entry of calcium ions into smooth muscle is the final common pathway which controls vasomotor tone, thus attenuating successive vasoconstrictor or vasodilator responses. Subsequent pilot and double-blind studies with these agents, e.g. flunarizine, nimodipine, verapamil, nifedipine, in adults have shown benefit (Louis and Spierings, 1982; Rascol *et al.*, 1986). Unwanted effects include nausea, abdominal pain, irritability, drowsiness, weight gain and hypotension. Calcium-channel blockers should not be used in the presence of renal, cardiovascular or hepatic disease. In classical migraine optimal relief of aura symptoms may be delayed for 10–14 days, and of headache for 2–4 weeks (Amery, 1983; Meyer and Hardenberg, 1983). The same studies have shown less good effect in common migraine, and frequent drug intolerance (e.g. in 37% of patients given verapamil, and 42% given nifedipine). It has been found that nimodipine may be the most effective, having more specific action, fewer side-effects, and better tolerance than flunarizine, verapamil and nifedipine (Gelmers, 1983; Meyer, 1985).

There have been few studies in children, mainly of flunarizine. In an open study Ferriere (1985) considered flunarizine was effective in 12 of 14 children, again noting that effectiveness developed gradually over 3 months. Sorge and Marano (1985) carried out a blind study on 48 children, of whom 24 were treated with flunarizine 5 mg and 24 with placebo. The flunarizine-treated children obtained a 60% reduction of frequency and 51% reduction in duration of headaches, whereas the placebo-treated group obtained a 32% and 16% reduction respectively. Unfortunately, only five of the children had classical migraine. There is a need for a properly conducted crossover trial of nimodipine and placebo in childhood migraine. It will be difficult to assess the effect of this agent on auras because of the variable frequency of auras in children with classical migraine, and, because of the long residual effect of calcium-channel blockers, it will be important to allow a 'washout' period of at least 1 month. An important study of the effect of flunarizine in the alternating hemiplegia syndrome, following a report of its efficacy in one child by Casaer and Azou (1984), illustrates some of the difficulties encountered in assessment of calcium-channel blockers (Caers *et al.*, 1987).

Antiepileptic drugs
Antiepileptic medication is sometimes recommended for the prophylaxis of childhood migraine (Prensky, 1976; Millichap, 1978; Barlow, 1984). It has been suggested that anticonvulsant drugs are more effective in children with 'paroxysmal electroencephalograms' (Froelich *et al.*, 1960). Prensky (1976) however reported that in his experience anticonvulsants were reasonably effective regardless of electroencephalographic findings. Phenobarbitone 30 mg twice daily or phenytoin 100–150 mg daily were recommended by Salmon (1977) and Barlow (1984). Maratos and Wilkinson (1982) reported that their most commonly used scheme of prevention of migraine in childhood was the daily administration of phenytoin. Our own experience with 110 children treated with phenobarbitone has however led us to the conclusion that double-blind trials will be essential to assess the value of antiepileptic drugs (particularly in relation to their side-effects) in the prophylaxis of childhood migraine. Such assessment will have to take into account the increasing understanding of the sometimes subtle effects of antiepileptic drugs on learning and behaviour (Hirtz and Nelson, 1985).

Alternative treatments
If dietary restriction or drug therapy in childhood migraine is as successful as some authors claim (Egger *et al.*, 1983: 93%; Barlow, 1984: 80%), it is surprising that so much interest is taken (particularly in the USA) in alternative methods of treatment. The problem with most of these is that: (1) they cannot be subjected to properly conducted double-blind controlled trials, and (2) many of them are time consuming and not readily available in hospitals in the UK.

Acupuncture   Most work in this field has been in adult migraine. Kajdos (1975) reported that headaches were relieved after 8–10 sessions in 136 of 304 patients, and Lenhard *et al.* (1983) in a study of 16 adults found a significant change in frequency and duration of headaches in 40%. Loh *et al.* (1984) in a double-blind study of 29 adults with acupuncture versus drug therapy found that a larger proportion preferred acupuncture. However, they acknowledged that their technique of acupuncture was time consuming for the doctor and painful for the patient – this, and the fact that acupuncture may have to be repeated several times, should be sufficient reason to restrict its use in children.

Biofeedback and relaxation therapy   During an investigation of the effects of autosuggestion on peripheral vasculature, a volunteer who happened to have a migraine observed that her attack improved as her hand temperature rose 10°F in 2 min (Sargent *et al.*, 1973). Subsequent studies using biofeedback to raise hand temperature or to constrict the temporal artery showed that migraine attacks could be aborted or their intensity diminished considerably. For an example, in an uncontrolled study Werder and Sargent (1984) observed reduction of migraine (and tension headache) in children aged 7–17 years, and also reduction in drug usage. The mechanism by which raising hand temperature, or constricting the temporal artery, might ameliorate the attack is not clear. With hand warming the patient is being conditioned to 'turn off' excessive sympathetic action, whereas with temporal artery constriction increased sympathetic activity is required. In an extensive review of the literature of relaxation and biofeedback therapy for adult migraine, Jessup *et al.* (1979) stated that studies so far were characterized by lack of either no treatment or placebo controlled groups, and by too small sample sizes, thus preventing reasonable conclusions about efficiency. In conclusion, they stated that controlled research on hand warming biofeedback, with or without relaxation, fails to support the specific benefit of these treatments for reducing migraine symptoms in adults. A critical review of the benefit of biofeedback in tension headache reached the same conclusion (*Lancet*, 1980). In a further review Holmes and Burish (1983) stated that there was no statistically reliable evidence from controlled studies that finger temperature biofeedback or temporal pulse amplitude biofeedback is effective in adult migraine.

Labbé and Williamson (1984), using a controlled group outcome design on 28 childhood migraine subjects aged 7–16 years, stated that 93% of the children treated by autogenic biofeedback for 7 weeks plus 1 month follow-up were significantly improved, i.e. 50% reduction of headaches, compared to no improvement in the control group. In a study of 18 children, aged 8–12 years old (Fentress *et al.*, 1986), six received frontal electromyographic biofeedback, meditative relaxation training and pain behaviour management, six meditative relaxation training and pain behaviour management without biofeedback, and the remaining six no treatment, for 11 weeks. The two treated groups experienced a significant reduction in headache symptoms compared to the children who received no treatment. Treatment was continued for the two treated groups for a year and it was found that there was no significant difference between them. These two trials on children suffer from the same drawbacks as identified by Jessup *et al.* (1979). The definition of migraine in the second study would not exclude children with tension headaches. Further controlled trials with adequate numbers of children and treated for a sufficient length of time are necessary in order to assess the value of biofeedback and relaxation therapy in childhood migraine.

Hypnotherapy   There are few reports of the value of hypnotherapy in adults (Hartland, 1966, 1971; Anderson *et al.*, 1975). There has been no published controlled study of the place of hypnotherapy in childhood migraine.

Prognosis

Although it is thought that childhood migraine has a better prognosis than adult migraine, there is little information about the latter in the literature (Whitty and Hockaday, 1968; Blau, 1987). Both of these studies were retrospective and, as Bille (1982) showed in his follow-up study, patients' memories are unreliable.

We are fortunate that Bille (1962) has continued to follow the 143 children included in his thesis for 25 years and 70 for 30 years. He divided them into two groups: (a) 73 with 'more pronounced' migraine and (b) 70 children with 'moderate migraine'. On follow-up of the former group 34–41% were free of migraine and of the latter group 51% were free of migraine (Bille, 1962, 1982). Other studies of childhood migraine have shown a 19–33% remission rate (Hinrichs and Keith, 1965; Koch and Melchior, 1969). In a study of 86 patients with onset of migraine before 16, eight relapsed after a 4-year remission and two after a 10-year remission (Hockaday, 1978), thus emphasizing the importance of at least a 10-year follow-up. In a 12-year follow-up of 108 children with migraine 34% obtained a complete remission (Congdon and Forsythe, 1979). It was suggested from this study that remissions were less likely to occur after 18 years, but between 7 and 17 years, 3–14% per annum obtain a complete remission. In a further follow-up of the 108 children, plus an additional 142 children followed for 12–20 years, 97 (39%) obtained a 12-year remission or longer, and 51 obtained remissions for 1–9 years before relapsing. Overall, approximately 30–40% of children with migraine may have a spontaneous remission lasting longer than 10 years. For futher comment on prognosis see Chapter 1.

Conclusion

Most children respond to reassurance, general advice, and simple remedies for treatment of attacks as they arise. An appropriate analgesic taken early in the attack, and a brief rest in a darkened room, are usually adequate. Prophylactic medication is indicated only for children with severe and frequent attacks (40% of cases in the first author's series), or in special circumstances. Prophylactic treatment for children is far from satisfactory, and the search for new and effective remedies must continue. In further studies much more careful attention needs to be given to defining subtypes of migraine, and new drugs must be subjected to rigorous double-blind comparisons with existing remedies, placebo treatment, and, most importantly, no treatment beyond explanation, reassurance, and appropriate management of acute attacks.

Chapter 6

Paroxysmal disorders which may be migraine or may be confused with it

Thierry W. Deonna

Introduction

When a child presents with paroxysmal and recurrent neurological symptoms of a more or less stereotyped nature and with no evident cause, unusual forms of epilepsy or migraine are usually the main possibilities considered. This is because these two conditions can cause virtually any type of paroxysmal neurological disorder and vegetative symptom, alone or in combination. The time-course of the deficit, the occurrence of more definite epileptic symptoms in some attacks, the presence of epileptic discharges on the EEG and the response to antiepileptic drugs usually, but not always, allow confirmation or exclusion of the diagnosis of epilepsy. The arguments for suspecting migraine in such situations are usually based on one or more of the following observations:

1. There is complete recovery of the deficit and no permanent handicap between episodes and no external cause or specific disease is identified.
2. Autonomic symptoms always or sometimes accompany the transient neurological or sensory symptoms.
3. There is a family history of a similar syndrome in a parent or a sibling.
4. There is a family history of migraine.
5. The child also has paroxysmal symptoms more closely resembling or typical of migraine attacks.
6. At follow-up the child develops symptoms typical of migraine.

None of these arguments is a proof that the disorder in question is in fact an atypical manifestation of migraine. It could be only a coincidence of two disorders, a rare one and a frequent one (migraine). Other features of the disorder may be more suggestive that it is in fact an alternative expression or an early manifestation of migraine:

1. The child always has migrainous symptoms as part of the attacks, even though they are not the main or the first complaint.
2. There is an adjunction of new migrainous symptoms as the disorder recurs.
3. The attacks alternate with typical migrainous attacks.
4. The disorder has never been seen without a family or personal history of migraine.
5. The child always develops migraine at follow-up.

Needless to say none of the disorders to be reviewed in this chapter meets these requirements. If so, there would be no discussion or need for it in the first place.

It must be remembered that a sudden neurological dysfunction or insult to the brain of any cause can trigger an attack of migraine in a susceptible patient. For example, a mild head trauma can trigger a severe migraine attack (and this tendency is sometimes very specific in certain families) or an epileptic child can have severe migraine-like headache after each seizure. Migraine is here only a 'complication' or a secondary symptom (but sometimes the most disturbing) of an aetiologically unrelated recurrent cerebral dysfunction. It is also well known that patients who develop progressive organic brain disorder (tumour, cyst, subdural haematoma) can have headaches of a typical migrainous character, if they are genetically predisposed or have already been suffering from migraine. Finally, there are numerous paediatric disorders where recurrent digestive symptoms are prominent (abdominal pain, nausea, vomiting) and can resemble migraine (Deonna, 1978). The basic disorder responsible for these symptoms may also trigger a migraine attack in a susceptible individual, so that closely related symptoms but of different origin and mechanism can coexist. For example, some inherited metabolic disorders can initially present with recurrent vomiting as the main symptom, usually precipitated by a stress (protein food excess, infection, accident, drugs). The similarity of these non-specific symptoms to some attacks of migraine does not mean an aetiological link, although it is possible that toxic metabolites can initiate a migraine attack.

Benign paroxysmal torticollis in infancy and benign paroxysmal vertigo of childhood

These two disorders are discussed together because both have been proposed as possible early forms of migraine and because their postulated mechanisms, clinical symptoms and evolution share many common features.

Benign paroxysmal torticollis in infancy

This disorder was first described by Snyder in 1969. Recurrent episodes of head tilt (torticollis) to the same or to the opposite side are noted in the first months of life. The abnormal head posture is the cardinal or the only sign, but a bent trunk posture (tortipelvis) may be present also (Chutorian, 1974). The onset may be as early as, or even before, the first month of life, but more often between the second and eighth month. An astonishing fact is the quite regular recurrence of the torticollis (about once a month) until it gradually disappears after a few months to a few years (1–5 years). There is usually no, or sometimes a non-specific precipitating factor. Usually, the parents have no warning that an attack is going to come. It seems to start in the morning in 90% of the cases (Hanakoglu et al., 1984). The torticollis lasts from a few hours to a few days.

During the attack, the head can be brought back to the vertical position but the infant puts it back immediately in the bent position and occasionally resents the manoeuvre (Militerni et al., 1983) although there is no visible spasm, tightness or pain in the neck muscles. Beside the torticollis, other associated symptoms are seen in the majority of the attacks:

1. Non-specific symptoms: irritability, drowsiness, 'unwell'.
2. Neurovegetative symptoms: pallor, redness, perspiration, headaches (in older children).
3. Signs of dysequilibrium or vestibular disturbance: refusal to walk, unsteady gait, and very rarely a transient nystagmus (Deonna and Martin, 1981).

It should be stressed that these symptoms can be entirely absent and the child can appear perfectly well apart from torticollis. At the opposite extreme, these symptoms can be very prominent and the torticollis may not even be mentioned by the parents. In a personal case (unpublished), the mother clearly distinguished two types of episodes: one with torticollis only, and the other with severe distress (screaming, redness of the face, vomiting, torticollis and tortipelvis). The neurological examination is normal during the attack (except for transient nystagmus and unsteadiness of gait if the child is already walking). The neuroradiological and electroencephalographic studies have always been negative.

The nature of the paroxysmal dysfunction responsible for BPT is unknown. Originally, Snyder (1969) proposed that a peripheral labyrinthine disturbance was the cause of the syndrome, because he found that the ice-water caloric test failed to produce nystagmus in the majority of the cases, and also because some children had a hypoacusis. However, his findings could not be confirmed in subsequent reports and no evidence of peripheral pathology in the vestibular or auditory system has been conclusively shown. A paroxysmal dysfunction of the central vestibular structures or their connections (as in BAM) could explain the majority of the observed symptoms and signs, although there is little direct evidence to support it (Sanner and Bergstrom, 1979). In a single case, M. Weissert (1987, personal communication) found an area of reduced perfusion during an attack of BPT in the cerebellar region on the side of the torticollis (using an intravenous labelled tracer: $^{99}Tc^m$-hexamethyl-propylenamin-oxim). A repeated examination done 2 weeks later in an asymptomatic period was normal. These data suggest that a transient vascular disturbance in the posterior fossa could account for these symptoms but these results need to be confirmed.

At the first attack, a number of diagnostic possibilities must be envisaged. Painful muscle spasm, or an acquired osteoarticular pathology of the craniocervical junction or of the neck must be ruled out, which is not always easy in an infant, especially when the baby is very irritable. A compensatory torticollis related to a cerebral, ocular (Raab and Snyder, 1970) or vestibular dysfunction must be considered. The most worrying diagnostic possibility is a posterior fossa or brainstem tumour. The acute onset, rapid recovery, and the absence of neurological signs except for a possible ataxia argue against this possibility. Abnormal head postures and movements can also be seen in cases of gastro-oesophageal reflux, oesophagitis, hiatus hernia or other pathology of the digestive system as has been reported under the name of Sandifer syndrome (Bray et al., 1977; Werlin et al., 1980). A dystonic drug reaction can affect mainly the neck muscles and cause an abnormal head posture (Casteels-Van Daele, 1979, 1982). Each of these entities has to be considered when taking the history or during observation of the child. Depending on when the child is first seen, and which symptoms are then still present or insisted upon by the parents, only further examination early in the course of a repeated attack will allow firm diagnosis.

How does review of the literature actually support the relationship between BPT and migraine? Between 50% and 60% of children with BPT show neurovegetative symptoms (mainly vomiting) and ataxia or unsteadiness of gait during the attacks. In contrast, a minority of children with BPT (10–20%) have been reported to have a history of headache or a family history of migraine (Hanakoglu *et al.*, 1984) or BPT (Lipson and Robertson, 1978; Sanner and Bergstrom, 1979) and only rare cases had documented attacks of migraine at follow-up. The absence of any mention of the family history in the early reports (Snyder, 1969), the difficulty of recording headache in the young child, and the brief duration of follow-up in the majority of cases make it difficult to come to a conclusion about the incidence of associated migraine in BPT. Well-documented cases have developed classical migraine, after the torticollis has subsided: that is, as the child grows the torticollis becomes gradually less but the associated symptoms (headache and vomiting) become the dominant complaint of the attack, which the parents recognize as the same basic disorder (Deonna and Martin, 1981; Menkes, 1985). The occurrence of attacks with and without associated neurovegetative symptoms in the same child (O. Bajc and S.Bajc, 1987, personal communication; personal observation) suggest that torticollis is only the most visible, the earliest and at times the only manifestation of the same basic syndrome. The great variability in the amount of autonomic symptoms and headache in children with definite migraine accompagnée may apply as well to BPT.

The limited number of reported cases of BPT so far, and the lack of clinical details and short follow-up in most cases do not at present allow a conclusion about how strong the relationship of this strange syndrome is to migraine. However, sufficient clinical arguments have already been accumulated to pursue the hypothesis that BPT is an early form of migraine. Dunn and Snyder (1976) reported children with BPT who later developed BPV which is also thought to be a possible early migraine equivalent (see below).

Further scrutiny of all clinical details of the personal and family history suggestive of migraine and study of the various features of individual attacks and their modification over a sufficient length of evolution in the same child and the differences between individual children is justified. This could help establish whether these are variations of the same basic disorder, or whether different aetiologies could account for the syndrome of BPT. It should be stressed that the diagnosis of BPT is not only a diagnosis of exclusion, but requires a search for associated symptoms suggestive of migraine. However, a positive family history of migraine is not an important, or safe, pointer to diagnosis at the onset of the disorder.

Treatment, if at all necessary, can of course be symptomatic only. It should be directed to what appear to be the most distressing features of the attack (vomiting, vertigo, headache). Because of the variety of reported cases, the relative infrequency of attacks and the variability of the symptoms, a systematic drug trial would be very difficult. To our knowledge no report has been published so far on this point.

Benign paroxysmal vertigo of childhood

BPV was originally described by Basser in 1964 and the following reports of the next 20 years (Koenigsberger *et al.*, 1968; Dunn and Snyder, 1976; Koehler, 1980; Eeg-Olofsson *et al.*, 1982) have essentially confirmed his initial observations. It is characterized by very sudden and recurrent attacks of true vertigo starting in early childhood. The onset is most often between 2 and 5 years, but cases starting before the age of 1 year or as late as 12 years have been reported. The attacks are stereotyped, can be quite frequent initially (once a month usually but can be as frequent as several per week) then occur less and less often to disappear altogether after a few months or a few years. It may not be obvious at the first attack that the symptoms can be explained by, and are secondary to, a vertiginous sensation, but it is remarkable that when the children can talk they invariably refer to such a sensation ('it spins', etc.). Children with BPV suddenly stop all activities, appear frightened, do not want to move or be moved and refuse to stand. If the attack occurs while the child is standing or walking, he appears very unsteady. He may be pale, nauseated and vomit. The attack usually lasts a few seconds, rarely a few minutes and exceptionally a few hours. Consciousness is not altered. The child seems perfectly well as soon as the attack is over.

There is no obvious precipitating factor in most cases. Occasionally, the attack is triggered by a manoeuvre which stimulates the vestibular system: indeed, some of these children dislike being turned rapidly, or thrown up and down, and they do not enjoy roundabouts and swings. The behaviour of the child during the attack, the reported vertiginous sensation and the associated symptoms (nausea or vomiting, nystagmus, ataxia, desire to remain absolutely still and exacerbation of the vertigo by movement) resemble the symptoms described in adults with sudden vestibular dysfunction. Several studies of the vestibular and auditory function in these children have given conflicting results. Originally, Basser (1964) and later Köenigsberger et al. (1968) reported a peripheral vestibular hyporeactivity ('canal paresis') using caloric tests. These findings could not be confirmed in later reports using more modern techniques. In fact, no demonstrable pathology of the central or peripheral vestibular system has been conclusively demonstrated in BPV and its cause or causes remain unknown.

Of course, vertigo in children, as in adults, can be the presenting symptom of a peripheral or central vestibular disturbance due to various diseases and requires a systematic differential diagnosis. The brief duration of the vertigo, after which the child immediately feels well and is normal on neurological examination, is unlike the vertigo associated with an acquired peripheral or central vestibular disturbance (i.e. vestibular neuronitis, posterior fossa inflammation or tumour).

Recurrent vertigo can be a specific epileptic symptom and it can be a prominent feature of an attack of migraine. Recurrent vertigo appears to be rare as a manifestation of childhood epilepsy (Beddoe, 1977; Blayney and Colman, 1984). In a single study (Eviatar and Eviatar, 1977), recurrent vertigo in children was found to be due to epilepsy in more than 50% of the cases. However, the data supporting the diagnosis of epilepsy in this study are not convincing. In contrast, recurrent vertigo is a frequent, and sometimes the most prominent, feature of migraine both in children (Watson and Steele, 1974; Verceletto et al., 1979) and in adults (McCann, 1982). Twenty-three of the 66 migrainous children studied by Watson and Steele (1974) had attacks of vertigo without headache. It thus seems that isolated recurrent vertigo can be a migraine equivalent in children. This of course raises the question whether BPV can be an early form of migraine. This was first proposed by Fenichel in 1967: he reported a child with typical BPV who later developed attacks with nausea, vomiting and headache in addition to the vertigo. The brother also had BPV and the mother suffered migraine headaches. The number of children with BPV who subsequently developed migraine or have a family history of migraine varies according to the reports from almost none to 80%. This probably reflects the bias of the authors or the mode of selection of the cases.

The sudden onset, brief duration, immediate recovery and the frequent absence of signs or symptoms other than those which can be directly related to the vertigo is striking in many of the reported cases of BPV and is unlike what is seen with migraine. Only one group of authors have recently claimed to have demonstrated that BPV is an early manifestation of migraine (Mira *et al.*, 1984; Lanzi *et al.*, 1986).

Mira *et al.* (1984) reported 13 children with BPV; eight of 13 had migraine or motion sickness and five and three respectively had cyclic vomiting and abdominal pain. They used headache provocation tests (nitroglycerine, histamine, fenflur-amine) which were positive in nine children and induced a vertigo in four children. The follow-up of these children was short (3–16 months) and it is not clear if the attacks of BPV were actually replaced by typical migraine. The same group (Lanzi *et al.*, 1986) published an almost identical paper 2 years later with the same conclusion but more patients. It was not specified if these were all new patients and there was no further detailed follow-up. There is no proof that the occurrence of headaches or vertigo after taking the above-named drugs is diagnostic of migraine. It is a frequent and probably non-specific reaction. Thus the data presented by these workers does not offer any new conclusive evidence about the relationship between BPV and migraine.

The striking variability in the age of onset, frequency and duration of the attack, age at remission, and the presence of associated symptoms in addition to the possible role of provoking factors (vestibular stimulation) together raise the possibility of different aetiologies within the syndrome of BPV. A positive family history of migraine or BPV, and the development of migraine in a few children who had BPV is only suggestive, but not proof, that BPV is an early equivalent of migraine. Again, the description of each individual attack in the same child, the evolution of the symptomatology and the modifications with age are all important features which should be documented, in order to further our understanding of the precise relationship between BPV and migraine. As far as treatment is concerned, the same remarks apply here for BPV as were made above for BPT.

Occipital epilepsy, basilar artery migraine and paroxysmal electroencephalographic abnormalities

When a child presents with transient visual disturbances and associated headaches, migraine is usually the first and only diagnosis considered. Positive visual phenomena (colours, lights, hallucinations, distortion of perception), or negative phenomena (loss or decrease of vision) can be reported by the child. The intensity of the headaches and autonomic signs and symptoms is quite variable. Epileptic discharges arising from the occipital or temporal cortex can also give rise to transient visual disturbances with or without associated epileptic symptoms and regardless of the nature of the underlying epileptic focus. If transient visual disturbances are the only manifestation of a seizure, differential diagnosis between migraine and epilepsy depends clinically on the rapidity of onset and disappearance of the visual symptoms and possibly also on their nature, although a description is often difficult to obtain, especially in young children.

In the last few years, a particular type of paroxysmal syndrome characterized by transient visual disturbances, severe associated migraine-like headaches and paroxysmal occipital spike-wave abnormalities has been reported. It was argued initially that these children suffer from a special type of basilar artery migraine and that the EEG discharges were secondary to repeated ischaemic episodes in the occipital lobes (Camfield *et al.*, 1978). Gastaut (1982) described a group of children with an identical symptomatology and EEG findings and proposed that they constituted a new epileptic syndrome akin to the benign focal epilepsy of childhood with Rolandic spikes and which he named 'benign focal epilepsy with occipital spike waves'. These children had transient visual disturbances of simple non-figurative type (impression of flashing lights, phosphenes, blurring of vision) of sudden onset and accompanied by severe headaches. The headaches were sometimes described as pulsatile with abdominal pain, nausea and vomiting, and indistinguishable from a migraine headache. The EEG showed biphasic spike-waves with a morphology and tendency to occur in clusters, as in the syndrome with Rolandic spikes, but located over one or both occipital regions. One striking characteristic of these spike-waves is that they are present only with the eyes closed and are immediately blocked on eye opening. They are not sensitive to photostimulation nor to hyperventilation. Opening and closure of the eyes in darkness (Panayiotopoulos, 1981) does not block the discharge as it does in light suggesting an inhibitory effect of central vision. The children reported by Gastaut (1982) had no neurological abnormalities, and had a normal CT scan, and there was a positive family history of epilepsy in 47% of the cases and of migraine in 19% of the cases. The seizures were easy to control, the course of the epilepsy was benign and the EEG abnormalities disappeared with age. Several arguments indicate that the syndrome initially reported by Camfield *et al.* (1978), and later by Gastaut (1982), and subsequently others, is primarily an epileptic disorder:

1. The onset and resolution of the visual disturbance is very rapid and more in keeping with an epileptic discharge than a migrainous phenomenon.
2. The visual disturbances may be followed by loss of consciousness, automatisms, or culminate in a hemiclonic or grand mal seizure indicating a propagation of the epileptic discharge.
3. The morphology and the behaviour of the spike-wave discharges are similar to those seen in benign focal epilepsy with Rolandic discharges and generalized spike-wave can be seen also.
4. The location of the discharge on the EEG can vary with age and may also be recorded more anteriorly in the centrotemporal regions (Herranz Tanarro *et al.*, 1984). This type of EEG abnormality is not seen with any frequency in complicated migraine nor, in particular, in BAM (Deonna *et al.*, 1984).

The specificity of this syndrome and its place among the 'benign' or 'functional' epilepsies of childhood should still be regarded as not entirely established for the following reasons:

1. Identical EEG abnormalities can be found in children who are evaluated because of a neurological handicap with or without epilepsy and with different types of seizures (Newton and Aicardi, 1983).
2. Some children continue to have seizures beyond adolescence; the benign course of the epilepsy has not been well established.
3. There is only a limited number of detailed reports of this syndrome and of sufficient follow-up.
4. The cause and the mechanisms of the headache and its possible relationship to migraine is not understood.

Further information on the following points would be important: the temporal profile and the nature of the visual phenomena that the children experience; the recording of an electroclinical seizure with all possible objective and subjective data occurring during that time. In our experience, it is difficult to have the children describe what they feel. The visual experience may be quite frightening and what the parents see may be described as a sudden panic which in fact could be the result of a sudden visual deprivation, especially in young children. Very recently, Kuzniecky and Rosenblatt (1987) reported a family in which three siblings had epilepsy and occipital spike-waves blocked by eye opening. A fourth sibling and the parents had EEG abnormalities but no seizures. No visual seizures were reported and only one had headache. These observations which will need to be expanded suggest a definite hereditary factor and an overlap between this syndrome and other genetically determined epilepsies, especially the 'benign focal epilepsy with Rolandic spikes'. It is thus reasonable at the present time to accept that there is a defined childhood epileptic syndrome which sometimes resembles and may be confused with, but is distinct from, migraine. The prognosis is probably good, but is not yet defined.

Post-traumatic syndromes and migraine

It is well recognized that trivial head trauma can be a precipitating factor of a migrainous attack. The classical example is that of footballer's migraine (Matthews, 1972), where the migraine attack follows shortly after a blow on the head from heading the ball.

The clinical manifestations of migraine following head trauma can be variable and it is probable that all forms of migraine (simple migraine or migraine with temporary neurological or behavioural symptoms) can be encountered. In some families, head trauma may be a regular and sometimes a specific trigger of the attacks (Haas et al., 1975). The reasons for attributing the transient neurological symptoms to migraine have been the following:

1. There is a close temporal relationship between the head trauma and migraine (usually 1–10 min).
2. There is usually a recurrence of similar symptoms after repeated trauma to the head.
3. The clinical features of the attack are indistinguishable from a spontaneously occurring migraine.
4. The child also has other spontaneous migrainous attacks.
5. There is a frequent family history of migraine.
6. There is a rapid complete recovery from the attack and no persisting symptoms suggesting a cerebral concussion and no laboratory evidence of a cerebral contusion.

Haas et al. (1975) have described four types of juvenile head trauma syndromes in which there are temporary neurological symptoms: somnolence irritability and vomiting; hemiparesis; blindness; brainstem signs. He, and later Guthkelch (1977), have offered good evidence that these syndromes are probably migraine variants; they are not mutually exclusive, and in fact are often associated (Haas and Lourie, 1984).

Two particular clinical syndromes deserve special discussion. (1) Transient blindness following head injury in children (Bodian, 1964; Griffith and Dodge, 1968): these children develop total transient blindness within minutes to a few hours following a seemingly trivial blunt head trauma. Restlessness and anxiety is prominent during the period of blindness but the behaviour rapidly returns to normal with recovery of vision. There are no abnormal ocular findings. If an EEG is done during the period of blindness, it shows bilateral occipital slowing. The cases reported by Greenblatt (1973) and later Haas et al. (1975) and Guthkelch (1977) clearly suggest that this syndrome is one of the possible transient neurological manifestations which can be attributed to migraine. (2) Special mention should be made of what has been called the 'delayed deterioration of consciousness after trivial head injury' (Haas and Lourie, 1984). It was initially thought to be due to post-traumatic brain oedema. Guthkelch (1977) has argued that the temporal profile of the disturbance is more in keeping with a vascular phenomenon than with brain oedema, and it has been suggested that stimulation of periaqueductal grey matter by a chemical mediator might reflexly alter cerebral blood flow, and thus account for the clinical picture (Bruce, 1984). This syndrome is probably a more severe form of the 'somnolence irritability and vomiting variant' described by Haas et al. (1975) and Menken (1978).

In a child with head trauma who develops progressive neurological symptoms and in whom a mass lesion can be excluded, the clinical course of the disorder must be carefully studied and other evidence of personal or family history of migraine must be looked for. It is very important not to attribute the neurological symptoms to the direct effect of trauma with all its possible medicolegal and psychological consequences, when other mechanisms such as migraine may be responsible.

Progressive disorders with paroxysmal neurological episodes resembling migraine

Alternating hemiplegia of childhood

This disorder is very rare and has been described in some detail in a limited number of publications (Verret and Steele, 1971; Hosking et al., 1978; Krägeloh and Aicardi, 1980). Recent interest and knowledge of this entity has developed following the observation of Casaer and Azou (1984) that flunarizine, a calcium entry blocker, completely aborted the attack in a child with this disease. A collaborative European study was then initiated by Casaer to study this drug in sufficient number of children, and the clinical picture of the disease has been discussed in several meetings. The first results of the drug study have just been published (Casaer, 1987).

The disorder starts very early in life (as early as 3 months and most often in the first 18 months) and is characterized by a sudden motor deficit affecting alternate sides of the body and lasting from a few hours to a few days, more rarely a few weeks. The motor deficit is not simply a hemiplegia as the name suggests (as in hemiplegic migraine or in postictal hemiplegia). Krägeloh and Aicardi (1980) have insisted on the presence of dystonic features: 'acute dystonia or tonic fits' on the affected side with loss of motor control. The limb(s) shows a sudden stiffening or takes an abnormal dystonic posture. Dittrich et al. (1979) also describe dystonic features. Head turning and tilting and ocular deviation can also be seen during the attack. Two other types of symptoms accompany the motor deficit:

1. Acute discomfort of the child variously described as 'misery', 'screaming', 'crying', 'irritability'.
2. Autonomic disturbances: pallor, vasomotor changes, paroxysmal respiratory irregularity.

The development of the child is normal until the onset of the attacks but a gradual deterioration is then seen over the next few years as the attacks continue. As the child gets older, the attacks become less frequent and severe and can cease altogether and the child is left with a chronic fixed deficit. All children develop a variable degree of mental handicap and signs of central motor disturbances. Dyskinesia (choreoathetosis) appears to be the most frequent sequel (as was seen in a personal case at age 24 years), but ataxia and hemiparesis have been reported. The cause of the disorder is a complete mystery. The hypothesis that the transient motor deficit is either an unusual seizure phenomenon or the result of a localized vascular insufficiency has never received any positive support from the numerous investigations that these children have undergone, both during attacks and in the free intervals (repeated EEGs and angiography). All attempts to treat these children with anticonvulsive or vasoactive drugs have been unsuccessful. The CT scan does not show any abnormality, either during the attacks or even at the stage of sequelae.

Verret and Steele (1971) initially proposed that AH was an early and severe form of complicated migraine. The eight children they reported had a positive family history of migraine; four out of eight had headaches as part of the attacks and two out of eight developed 'a more characteristic picture of migraine'. In the European collaborative study conducted by Casaer (1987), 50% had a history of migraine. The descriptions of the associated symptoms during the attacks of AH and the follow-up of the children do not often document the presence of headaches or other characteristics of migraine, either during or between the attacks. A striking decrease in the severity and the frequency of the attacks with flunarizine, a drug with many different properties (calcium entry blocking agent, modification of the arterial tone, etc.), has been documented in several cases of AH. The children who responded to the drug have so far not shown neurological deterioration provided treatment was started early in the course of the disease (Casaer, 1987). Also, the behaviour of the children and their general 'well being' was said to be very much improved: even if they still had attacks, these seemed to be much more tolerable. Flunarizine (Sibelium) has been found to be effective in controlled studies of adults with migraine (Louis, 1981). Preliminary reports of the use of this substance in children with migraine have also been positive (G. Chiamanti et al., personal communication, 1985). However, given the complex and diverse modes of action of this substance (Holmes et al., 1984), the finding of a beneficial effect of flunarizine both in AH and migraine (Lagreze et al., 1986) is not a definite argument for a common pathophysiology in the two disorders.

At the present time, AH should be regarded as a separate disorder with a unique set of symptoms and signs unlike other known paroxysmal disorders. There is no evident relationship with familial hemiplegic migraine in which attacks start at a much later age (8–10 years), there is complete recovery between the attacks, and no dyskinetic component of the motor disorder; the parents of these children also have migraine with hemiplegic attacks (Glista et al., 1975; Müller and Müller,

1977). Review of the cases reported as BAM in childhood (Golden and French, 1975; Hockaday, 1979; Ritz *et al.*, 1981) do not show a close relationship with AH despite the fact that many symptoms of AH can be attributed to brainstem dysfunction. Hockaday (1979) in a detailed paper on BAM discussed two atypical cases closely resembling AH which she clearly separated from the others. In summary, the main arguments for differentiating AH from migraine are:

1. It is a progressive disorder.
2. There is no family history with a sibling also affected with AH.
3. The incidence of a family or personal history in AH is variable according to the reports, and the maximum found (50%) is less than in typical migraine.
4. The paroxysmal motor disorder is not simply a hemiparesis as in migraine accompagnée.

Mitochondrial cytopathies

This is a recently recognized group of hereditary metabolic disorders affecting the function of various enzymes involved with energy metabolism in the mitochondria (Petty *et al.*, 1986). The mitochondrial abnormalities were first recognized in the muscle biopsy (the so-called ragged red fibres; morphological abnormalities of the mitochondria are seen on electron microscopy). The three main recognized clinical types of these disorders are:

KSS syndrome — the Kearns–Sayre syndrome: progressive ophthalmoplegia, signs of CNS involvement, muscle weakness, visceral involvement and growth failure.

MERRF syndrome — the Myoclonic Epilepsy–Ragged Red Fibre syndrome.

MELAS syndrome — the Mitochondrial myopathy and Encephalopathy with Lactic Acidosis and Stroke-like episodes syndrome (Pavlakis *et al.*, 1984).

The MELAS syndrome can initially present with acute and transient hemiplegia associated with headaches and vomiting, and the diagnosis of migraine may be suspected in these cases early in their course, before the progressive neurological deterioration occurs. The development of the child is normal before the onset of the disease, usually in the first 10 years of life. Transient neurological deficits such as cortical blindness, recurrent and alternating hemiplegia or hemianopia have been seen in the course of the disease (F. Goutière and G. Ferrière, 1986, personal communication). Growth failure, muscle weakness, pyramidal, extrapyramidal and cerebellar signs, and cortical blindness have been described as the disease progresses. The diagnosis can be made on the basis of a lactic acidosis and ragged red fibres on the muscle biopsy. A mitochondrial enzyme deficiency is likely, but the exact defect(s) has not been found yet. The CT scan is abnormal in all cases but not specific: basal ganglia calcifications, cortical atrophy, occipital (and other) hypodensities have all been described (Hasuo *et al.*, 1987). If a child presents with a transient neurological disorder of undefined nature suggesting a cerebral ischaemic episode, with a prolonged course, incomplete recovery, and especially if he has a growth deficiency and abnormal neurological development, the MELAS syndrome should be suspected. A lactic acidosis and ragged red fibres in the muscle biopsy have been found in all cases of MELAS so that this diagnosis can be confirmed or ruled out with these data (F. Goutière and G. Ferrière, 1986, Personal Communication).

Inherited disorder of urea cycle metabolism: hyperammonaemia due to ornithine transcarbamylase deficiency (OTC) and migraine

Repeated severe vomiting with or without lethargy and confusion can be an important symptom of some inherited metabolic disorders, particularly those of the urea cycle resulting in hyperammonaemia. Hyperammonaemia can be precipitated by various stresses: infection, trauma, and (mainly) excessive protein intake. Cyclical vomiting is in some cases an early 'migraine equivalent'. It has thus been thought that cyclical vomiting could be a manifestation of an underlying inherited metabolic abnormality precipitated by some endogenous intermittent intoxication. Russell (1973) was the first to propose that severe migraine could also be a manifestation of the heterozygous state of OTC deficiency, due to an inability to handle an excess of ammonia. He described two mothers with children affected with OTC deficiency. The two mothers had a family and a personal history of migraine and had intense attacks of migraine following an ammonia tolerance test. He also found that nine of 15 well-defined cases of juvenile migraine had an abnormally high fasting blood ammonia level.

Following Russell's original paper (1973), we have not found any well-documented report showing a similar close association between migraine and OTC deficiency (de Bruijn et al., 1976). In fact, a computer-based literature search for the past 20 years gave only two papers on this topic (de Bruijn et al., 1976; Gilchrist and Coleman, 1987). Rowe et al. (1986) did not observe headache in their detailed study of 13 symptomatic females with OTC deficiency. Recently, C. Bachmann (personal communication, 1987) studied 26 cases of OTC deficiency seen in the past 10 years. None of his patients presented clinically with a history suggestive of migraine and the family history of migraine in his cases was not greater than that found in the normal population. Thus it is very likely that the earlier reported association of OTC deficiency and migraine was fortuitous. OTC deficiency must be considered in any patient with severe repeated vomiting, confusion, lethargy or behaviour disturbance of unknown cause, and it is thus an important differential diagnosis from migraine.

Summary

Peculiar childhood paroxysmal disorders which may be, or may be confused with, migraine have been reported in the past few years. Their aetiology, pathogenesis and nosological position is still unclear, but from the clinical point of view they constitute distinct clinical syndromes which need to be recognized for several reasons:

1. The cardinal signs or symptoms are not specific and can be seen in other more frequent neurological disorders from which they need to be distinguished.
2. The prognosis is often benign and a correct diagnosis early in the course is very important to avoid unnecessary examinations and anxiety.
3. The symptoms are very alarming and serious neurological diseases can be suspected.
4. Exceptionally, they can be the presenting signs of well-recognized progressive neurological disorders for some of which therapeutic possibilities do exist.

The features of these disorders which suggest they actually are or might be an 'equivalent' or early manifestation of migraine are the following: the child always has migrainous symptoms as part of the attacks, even though they are not the main or the first complaint; there is an adjunction of new migrainous symptoms as the disorder recurs; the attacks alternate with typical migrainous attacks; the disorder has never been seen without a family or personal history of migraine; the child always develops migraine at follow-up. Of course, none of the disorders reviewed in this chapter meets all these requirements.

Benign paroxysmal torticollis is characterized by repeated 'attacks' of torticollis to either side, starting usually before 6 months of life and disappearing after a few months to a few years. Autonomic symptoms and ataxia may or may not be associated during the attacks, which last from a few hours to a few days. In a minority of children with this syndrome, the attacks are gradually replaced by typical migrainous attacks. In *benign paroxysmal vertigo,* the child has repeated brief attacks of intense true vertigo lasting a few seconds and rarely minutes or hours, after which recovery is immediate and complete. If the child can not yet describe the symptoms, one has to rely on the overall dynamics of the symptoms and associated behaviour of the child during the attack.

Occipital epilepsy, intercalated migraine and paroxysmal EEG abnormalities is a curious, still incompletely defined, epileptic syndrome. The child has paroxysmal visual disturbances followed sometimes by other epileptic symptoms, often with severe headaches resembling migraine. The EEG shows paroxysmal discharges in the parieto-occipital regions blocked by eye opening. It is probably akin to the benign focal epilepsy of childhood with Rolandic spikes.

Trauma can be a specific or non-specific trigger of classical or complicated migraine attacks in predisposed individuals. Various migrainous *post-traumatic syndromes* have been described. The symptoms develop immediately or in the hours following head injury. *Transient cortical blindness* following head injury in children is a special and dramatic example and should be considered when a conscious but agitated child has no active visual responses after a minor head trauma. A precise diagnosis of these migrainous attacks precipitated by head trauma is important because the symptoms may be wrongly attributed to direct traumatic brain damage with all its negative psychological and medicolegal consequences.

In *alternating hemiplegia* of childhood, the child has repeated attacks of unilateral motor deficit (weakness, dystonic postures) accompanied by autonomic disturbance lasting from a few hours to a few days and starting very early in life (3–18 months). Over the years, the child becomes retarded with a fixed central motor deficit. This rare disorder was thought to be a severe form of 'migraine accompagnée' but recent data indicates that it is a separate disorder of unknown aetiology with no certain relation to migraine. Renewed interest in this rare syndrome had followed the observation that flunarizine can suppress the attacks and possibly prevent the progression of the disorder in some children, whereas prior to this all forms of treatment had been unsuccessful.

Among the mitochondrial cytopathies, the *MELAS syndrome* can start with stroke-like reversible deficits, resembling 'migraine accompagnée'.

Recurrent vomiting, somnolence, confusion and lethargy can follow infection, stress or excessive food intake in patients with hyperammonaemia due to ornithine transcarbamylase (OTC) deficiency, but there is no good evidence that this disorder can be a cause of, or has a close relationship with, typical migraine.

Chapter 7

Migraine and epilepsy

Judith M. Hockaday and Richard W. Newton

The most frequent relation of migraine to epilepsy is as a source of error. (Gowers 1907, p. 100)

The relationships between migraine and epilepsy are complex. Although most would now consider Gowers' dictum untrue, there are still areas of difficulty, uncertainty and controversy. The subject remains clinically important. This chapter will attempt to cover the clinical aspects and will refer only briefly to theoretical considerations. For these, reference should be made to specialist texts (e.g. Amery and Wauquier, 1986; Andermann and Lugaresi, 1987; Olesen and Edvinsson, 1988).

Because of the complexities, this discussion will be presented in relation to a series of special aspects:

The genetic relationship between migraine and epilepsy.
The electroencephalographic features of migraine.
Migraine as a cause of epilepsy.
Alteration of consciousness and seizures during attacks of migraine.
Acute confusional states, and prolonged coma in migraine.
Visual symptoms in migraine.
Childhood occipital epilepsy and 'intercalated migraine'.
Seizure headaches.

The genetic relationship between migraine and epilepsy

It has not been established that migraine and epilepsy have a common pathophysiology. Recent work suggests there may be a limited genetic link. Many early studies are open to criticism because they are retrospective, or are of selected patient groups. Whitty (1972) wrote: 'The edge of the statistical instrument is blunted if the diagnostic categories it assesses are . . . variable and imprecise'. This is the case in both epilepsy and migraine where what is inherited is not necessarily the disorder but the predisposition to it, and where epidemiological study may be marred by uncertain or arbitrary definition and inadequate or distorted recall. The many reports in the early literature claiming a higher incidence of epilepsy in patients with migraine must be judged in the light of the above difficulties. They should also be reassessed in the light of better understanding of the pathophysiology of migraine and of the mechanisms whereby consciousness may be altered or lost, or seizures occur, during migraine attacks. The early literature also needs reassessment in the light of better understanding of the variability of the EEG in childhood.

For example, in a review of the diagnosis and treatment of migraine in children Prensky and Sommer (1979) stated that their results 'agree with previous reports that epilepsy is present in more migrainous patients than in other children'. Nine of the 64 children in their series with migraine who had EEGs also had seizures, but the cases were highly selected, from a paediatric neurology service, and studied retrospectively. Moreover, not all of the seven 'previous reports' they cited would now be considered valid, and the others do not support the contention. In particular, the major study quoted, which was well controlled, and population based, by Bille (1962), did *not* find any evidence of an association between migraine and epilepsy in children. Again while Selby and Lance (1960) reported that as many as 11% of 348 patients with migraine had epilepsy, in the later report of their larger prospective study they found a lower incidence of epilepsy in the migraine group (1.6%) than in a control group of patients with tension headache (2%) (Lance and Anthony, 1966). As the authors pointed out, the relatively high incidence in both groups was to be expected in hospital referred case series. However, in a similarly controlled study Basser (1969) found the incidence of epilepsy significantly higher in 1830 patients with migraine (5.9%) than in 548 patients with tension headache (1.1%) ($P < 0.0005$). It is possible that a modifying factor in this analysis was the higher rate of 'unclassifiable loss or impairment of consciousness' in the tension headache (control) group.

There have been other negative studies. Lees and Watkins (1963), Slatter (1968) and Klee (1968) all found a low incidence of epilepsy (unassociated with the migraine attack) in large series (respectively six in 359, seven in 184, and five in 150, cases). Koch and Melchior (1969) found a low familial rate of epilepsy in both migraine and non-migraine headache, and Ziegler and Wong (1967) actually commented upon the absence of overt seizures in their study. In more recent childhood studies Congdon and Forsythe (1979) found nine of 300 children gave a history of epilepsy, while Barlow (1984) noted only five of his 300 cases had afebrile seizures unassociated with the migraine attack. Baier (1985) found a familial prevalence of convulsions in only 1.4% of 81 subjects with childhood onset migraine, this being less than the general epidemiological risk in his community. Kraus (1978) quoted extensively by Andermann and Andermann (1987) found the prevalence of migraine was similar among relatives of epileptic and control subjects.

There have been three recent studies of migraine in clinically selected and probably homogeneous subgroups of childhood epilepsy. In two the authors concluded that an association between migraine and epilepsy exists. Baier and Doose (1985) studied families of children with childhood absence epilepsy and found the risks of epilepsy and migraine were both higher in the relations of female than of male propositii, arguing a related 'genetic background'. Seshia *et al.* (1985) reported a higher than expected association between migraine and partial seizures with complex symptomatology. However, this study is to be criticized because the seizures are not defined according to current classification (Commission on Classification and Terminology, 1981) and in 74% of cases migraine was of common type: diagnosis of this can only be presumptive, and, in context, the distinction from 'seizure headache' is unclear (see below). The third study (Santucci *et al.*, 1985) found no evidence of a link between migraine and benign epilepsy with Rolandic spikes.

Conclusion

In general, therefore, the evidence is against a common genetic background (or common pathophysiology) of migraine and epilepsy. (For further comment see Chapter 2.)

It follows that in clinical practice where migraine and epilepsy both occur in the same child, the association should be regarded as fortuitous: each disorder should be considered on its own merits, and investigated and treated accordingly.

Electroencephalographic changes in migraine

Changes in the EEG between, and during, attacks of migraine, in resting state recordings and in responses to stimuli, have been known for a long time. Parsonage (1975) summarized the main findings as: focal and generalized slow waves, spike-wave discharges, local spike- or sharp-waves, abnormal hyperventilation responses, and an extended range of response to flicker. Most earlier observations were interictal in selected uncontrolled case groups. The subject has been reviewed recently by Hockaday and Debney (1988).

Interpretation of the EEG and understanding of what is normal, especially in younger ages, has altered in recent years, in a way suggesting that many earlier studies may have overestimated the number of records considered abnormal. Kinast *et al.* (1982) refer to some of the features which would now be accepted as normal: prominent posterior slowing, polyphasic potentials, rhythmic posterior slow, hypnogogic hypersynchrony, 6-Hz phantom spike-and-wave, psychomotor variant, and 'small sharp spikes', all these now being considered as normal patterns but frequently interpreted as abnormal in previous studies.

Interictal changes

All studies have agreed in finding no change specific for migraine and, again in all studies, a proportion of EEGs was considered normal. It is likely that the changes known, and repeatedly confirmed, are another expression of the underlying constitutional predisposition to migraine, rather than a specific association or result of migraine attacks. The variation in earlier findings in children is shown by the following two reports. In a hospital-based study Prensky and Sommer (1979) found the EEG normal in only 27% of children, the remainder showing diffuse slowing, sharp waves, paroxysmal changes and focal abnormalities. In contrast, in a population study in schoolchildren, Bille (1962), using case-matched controls, observed abnormal records in only 22% of children with pronounced migraine – and while abnormality in the control group was less (15%) the difference did not reach significance. However, he did note that while both the migraine subjects and the controls experienced subjective disturbances during photic stimulation equally (45%), headache was provoked more often in the migraine group. Furthermore, analysis of responses to photic stimulation showed a significantly greater incidence of driving at fast frequencies in the migraine group, in line with the earlier observations of Golla and Winter (1959). In another recent study of 100 children with migraine, Kinast *et al.* (1982) also found the great majority (89%) of EEG recordings normal. However, they reported sharp waves 'characteristic of benign focal epileptic discharges of childhood' as the only feature in nine of the 11 abnormal records. This incidence is significantly higher than the 1.9% found in healthy schoolchildren by Eeg-Olofsson et al. (1971). The interpretation of this is difficult, as 15% of children in the migraine study had a history either of febrile convulsions or familial epilepsy.

More recent studies have used quantitative analysis of the resting interictal EEG. Jonkman and Lelieveld (1981) used EEG computer analysis to study 20 control-matched migraine subjects (13 'classic', seven common) and found four parameters (including variations of alpha power and frequency, and responses to photic stimulation) which characterized 55% of the migraine group compared to only 5% of the control group. Abnormality was visually identified in a further four cases (20%) (sharp waves, spike wave complexes, or abnormal hyperventilation responses).

It is unlikely that the changes noted in the interictal EEG are the direct result of the effects of attacks, except in rare instances (Slatter, 1968; see below). Hockaday and Whitty (1969) found no tendency for a higher incidence of EEG abnormality in patients with a long history of frequent attacks than in those with a short history of infrequent attacks, nor in those with severe as opposed to mild symptoms, and lateralized interictal abnormality 'marking' a stereotyped consistently lateralized aura was seen as often in subjects with a short history of infrequent attacks as in those with a long history of frequent attacks. The changes observed by Jonkman and Lelieveld (1981) were also not related either to headache frequency or duration of the disorder. However, Smyth and Winter (1964) related some EEG changes to duration of the disorder, while Klee (1968) found the EEG more often abnormal with high overall attack severity than with low severity. And in a later study of the long-term outcome of childhood-onset migraine, Hockaday (1978) found that while the majority of EEG records became (or remained) normal at review, a small number (10%) became abnormal, and in one case (of 29 studied serially) localization of 'dysrhythmic' abnormality appropriate to the site of the aura appeared as a new feature, possibly reflecting permanent damage.

Ictal changes

Most reports of EEG changes during migraine attacks describe transient slow wave disturbance in classical migraine, diffuse or focal according to the aura, and reflecting the local neuronal abnormality. Studies have been made in hemiplegic migraine (reviewed by Bradshaw and Parsons (1965), Harding et al. (1977), classical migraine with non-visual aura (Rossi et al., 1980), BAM (Swanson and Vick, 1978), and migraine with impairment of consciousness (Walser and Isler, 1982)). 'Slow wave depression' has also been observed in ACM (discussed below), and in migrainous transient global amnesia (Sacquegna et al., 1985; see below).

There are fewer studies in common migraine but recently Puca et al. (1985) using EEG spectral analysis observed diffuse or focal delta or theta activity, or attenuation of alpha amplitude, during spontaneous (or drug-induced) attacks of both common and classical migraine. Schoenen et al. (1987) had similar findings in common migraine attacks: they reported transient alpha attenuation on the side of the headache in those with hemicrania. There was no correlation with severity, or duration of pain.

While most observations in BAM have been of transient slow wave disturbance, usually but not always posteriorly, Parain and Samson-Dollfus (1984) found that eight of nine cases did not show slow wave changes, but instead had transient diffuse predominantly frontal fast activity during the attacks. This variation was linked with the clinical expression of the attacks which were predominantly brainstem, and did not include visual disturbance. There are a number of reports of BAM with seizures and severe (epileptic) EEG abnormalities (Camfield *et al.*, 1978; Panayiotopoulos, 1980) and discussion of this syndrome in relation to occipital epilepsy in children (Deonna *et al.*, 1984). The feature in common in these reports is the presence of occipital spike-wave complexes suppressed by eye opening, and of seizures with transient loss of consciousness, sometimes with preceding visual loss/disturbance, and then headaches, nausea and vomiting, and thus close similarity to, and perhaps evolution to, migraine. This form of epilepsy and its clinical relationship with migraine is discussed below (see also Chapter 6).

Evoked response testing

It is likely that the higher than chance incidence of a PCR to IPS in migraine subjects reported in past literature is the result of bias in case referral and reporting (Hockaday and Debney, 1988). There appears to be no overlap between the clinical syndrome of light-sensitive epilepsy and visually induced migraine (Debney, 1984).

The significance of an increased incidence of photic driving (an induced rhythmical occipital response to IPS, itself a normal phenomenon) at fast frequencies repeatedly observed in migraine subjects is not clear. The findings in most studies are similar (e.g. Golla and Winter, 1959; Bille, 1962; Slatter, 1968; Friedman and Pampiglione, 1974), but not all studies are adequately controlled, nor do they allow for factors of anxiety and overarousal, known to be prominent in migraine. The special nature of the prominence of driving at fast frequencies of IPS may thus be only indirectly related to the migraine, and (like the changes in the resting EEG; see above) merely an expression of the underlying constitutional predisposition, showing itself as an overactive sympathetic nervous system.

The significance of the differences from normal found in evoked response studies is also not clear. Studies using visual (flash, and pattern reversal), auditory and somatosensory stimulation are difficult to interpret, because of variations in the populations studied, the methods used, and the (sometimes opposed) findings. In a well-controlled study by Gawel *et al.* (1983) significant differences in the form of the visually evoked potential in migraine and control subjects were found (confirming some earlier observations, e.g. Kennard *et al.*, 1978), and the authors postulate either a failure of sensory input modulation, or an abnormal response to input, the result of disturbed neurotransmitter function in the migraine subjects. Similar differences consisting of increased amplitude on flash (but not pattern) stimulus have been reported recently in children (Brinciotti *et al.*, 1986). The subject of evoked response abnormality in migraine is further discussed by Hockaday and Debney (1988).

Migraine as a cause of epilepsy

Alteration or loss of consciousness and other features suggesting epilepsy are well known to occur during attacks of migraine and have important implications for management (see Chapter 1: Symptomatic migraine, and below). The question here is whether ordinary non-symptomatic migraine can lead to the appearance of new (recurring) epilepsy where no susceptibility to epilepsy existed previously.

There is very little evidence of this even in patients known to have sustained permanent cerebral damage on clinical, radiological or EEG evidence. Case reports of complicated migraine, some in childhood, with persisting neurological abnormality, do not report epilepsy as a new feature (Connor, 1962; Bradshaw and Parsons, 1965; Ment *et al.*, 1980). Previous studies of migraine patients by CT scanning have reported lesions described as small infarcts, or focal or generalized atrophy (Hungerford *et al.*, 1976; Mathew *et al.*, 1977); many of the cases discussed had experienced frequently repeated hemiplegic migraine, but no new epilepsy emerged.

Similarly long-term follow-up studies do not describe an increasing incidence of epilepsy (Hinrichs and Keith, 1965; Whitty and Hockaday, 1968; Congdon and Forsythe, 1979). In a study of 40 childhood cases of complicated migraine, Rossi *et al.* (1980) observed one child with accompanying temporal lobe epilepsy, and two who showed clonic movements during attacks of hemiplegic migraine; in no patient did new epilepsy arise during follow-up to 15 years. Hockaday and Whitty (1969) found no greater incidence of epilepsy in patients with repeated unilateral aura always on the same side than in patients with aura arising from either side. Ziegler (1984) did not report epilepsy in a long-term follow-up study of 127 patients with migraine associated with neurological abnormality during attacks.

However, there are isolated case reports where epilepsy (or EEG epileptic activity) appears to have arisen as a result of severe migraine in the absence of pre-existing organic cause (for EEG change see above). Bickerstaff (1962) described an unheralded epileptic attack in a boy aged 17 years, several months after severe BAM. Barolin (1966) refers to six patients who 'developed epileptic fits after many years of severe migraine' in a group of 14 patients with migraine and epilepsy. Slatter (1968) described two patients in whom he considered that 'focal brain damage caused by migraine may have caused local epileptic change': one was a boy aged 8 years who developed status epilepticus and then grand mal epilepsy with a left occipital focus after frequent attacks of BAM. Perhaps the most convincing case report is that of Pearce and Foster (1965) who described Jacksonian epilepsy and then two major seizures in a 16-year-old girl with classical migraine and no demonstrable underlying lesion. These case histories suggest that 'hypoxic-ischaemic' effects in the course of migraine might lead to neuronal damage and the establishment of spontaneous seizure activity.

Conclusion

The rarity of these cases must be emphasized. In general the occurrence of epileptic attacks, particularly if partial, in a patient with migraine headaches is a clear indication for investigation. Both Pearce and Foster (1965) and Slatter (1968) include in their studies cases where the migraine and epilepsy were symptomatic of cerebral angioma (see below and Chapter 1), and Barolin (1966) included in his series of migraine cases five where the paroxysmal headaches and epileptic fits were the common expression of cerebral tumour (two), vascular malformation (two) and 'contusio cerebri' (one).

Alteration of consciousness during migraine

There are a number of different ways in which consciousness may be altered or lost in migraine and also in which seizures may occur during attacks.

Liveing (1873) and Gowers (1907) classified migraine among the epilepsies. The work of Wolff (Dalessio, 1987a) led to concentration for a time on the purely vascular component of the attack. Bickerstaff (1961b) suggested that cerebral ischaemia in a potentially epileptic brain could account for some examples of loss of consciousness during migraine. More recently events have turned full circle with a model proposed of primary neuronal dysfunction of brainstem and hypothalamus (Pearce, 1984a; see Chapter 8). During an attack of migraine seizure activity in affected neurones could arise through primary perhaps genetically mediated factors within the cell or in response to an alteration in the cell environment. There may be changes in ionic content of the interstitium, the result perhaps of hypoxia due to local ischaemia or systemic hypoperfusion. Structural distortions of neurones and their vascular supply, for example by angioma, may be important in rare cases. It is possible that spreading cortical depression first described by Leão in 1944 underlies the aura of classical migraine (Lauritzen, 1986; Leão, 1986; see Chapter 8). During this, increased electrical activity occurs at the spreading edge of the depressed neuronal activity, and this could be a mechanism of seizure activity (Schadé, 1959).

Bickerstaff (1961b) suggested that transient brainstem ischaemia affecting the reticular formation could lead to impairment or loss of consciousness and also to the unusual deep sleep states sometimes seen in BAM. His description is worth quoting in full:

> the loss of consciousness (in BAM) was always curiously slow in onset – never abrupt, and never causing the patient to fall or be injured. A dreamlike state sometimes preceded unconsciousness. The degree of unconsciousness was never profound and the patients were never unrousable; on vigorous stimulation they could be aroused to good co-operation but they returned to unconsciousness when the stimulation ceased. (Bickerstaff, 1961b, p. 1058)

Lee and Lance (1977) proposed involvement of neurotransmitter pathways of the midbrain (linked with the reticular formation) as a possible 'single site' for the origin of the very prolonged loss of consciousness occasionally occurring in BAM attacks (migraine stupor). Lance et al. (1983) showed how the locus coeruleus may be part of an important intrinsic neural pathway allowing brainstem nuclei to affect the microcirculation of the cortical mantle.

The pain of migraine headache might act as a trigger for syncope in some, and genetic predisposition to an inherently high vagal tone could underly the susceptibility in others (Lombroso and Lerman, 1967; Stephenson, 1978).

From the foregoing it is clear that a number of different mechanisms may underlie alteration and loss of consciousness, feelings of faintness and seizures during migraine.

Fainting and loss of consciousness

It has been suggested that migraine subjects in general are more prone to fainting attacks due to orthostatic hypotension, quite independently of their migraine attacks. This was observed by Bille (1962) who found that 21 (29%) of 73 children with pronounced migraine (PMi) had symptoms of orthostatic insufficiency which included syncope in nine. It is not clear how often this was part of a migraine attack. It is noteworthy that Bille (1962) did not include syncope or alteration of consciousness as symptoms of the attack in the community school-based survey overall of 347 children with migraine – pointing perhaps to the rarity of these phenomena in ordinary migraine experience.

One study which looked only at patients experiencing loss of consciousness during the migraine attack found this rare (Lees and Watkins, 1963): in a retrospective analysis of 354 patients with migraine attending a neurology clinic (plus another five patients from an epileptic series), there were only 23 who experienced loss of consciousness during attacks. Six patients had migraine and epilepsy occurring separately. Of the remainder, the majority were patients with BAM (seven) with unconsciousness (plus incontinence in two) regarded as due to reticular anoxia, or patients described as experiencing syncope in the course of abortive BAM (six), or other forms (seven), leaving only three cases, all children, in which the nature of the loss of consciousness was regarded as epileptic – two showing rigidity and one a grand mal attack.

Lance and Anthony (1966) selected 500 patients with a migraine attack frequency at least once monthly from their prospective study of 1152 patients attending a neurological department headache clinic, and found 97 (19%) had experienced some impairment of consciousness as part of the attack. Feelings of faintness occurred in 38 and actual syncope, commonly at the height of the headache, in 23. Only two patients had one or more major epileptic seizures during attacks of migraine. The remaining 34 had experienced 'confusion, amnesia, automatisms, disorientation'. These features were very significantly linked with the occurrence of focal neurological symptoms. Fainting and feelings of faintness were commonly associated with the 'vertebrobasilar system' and confusional states with the 'carotid system' (by inference).

Barolin (1966) discussed the complex relationships between migraine and epilepsy in 15 patients showing paroxysmal headaches and 'epileptic signs' selected from 260 migraine patients attending a neurology department. In five cases the migraine was symptomatic (see above), in two migraine and epilepsy occurred independently and in two a migraine attack culminated in a seizure. In the remaining six patients severe migraine was considered to have led to the development of epilepsy many years later. 'Syncopal faints also occurred.' The incidence of syncope overall – sometimes linked with the migraine attack, sometimes independent – in the series was 13%. He described one case in detail that was of particular interest: a 25-year-old female typist with episodes of vertical headache of sudden onset, lasting several hours, sometimes with associated vomiting, from the age of 16. Attacks occurred once or twice monthly and once or twice a year she would faint in an attack, usually after some hours of headache. She would have a 'syncopal aura' (sic) and then slump toneless and pale without convulsive movement. A dysrhythmic EEG was treated with anticonvulsants but the bouts were unaltered. An EEG with ocular compression showed 4.5 s of asystole reflecting an inherently high vagal tone. For 11 months she succeeded in aborting attacks by taking ergotamine, caffeine and an antihistamine. She then had three seizures, in which she smiled inappropriately, and showed deviation of the eyes, loss of awareness and repetition of stereotyped words. These complex partial seizures then became secondarily generalized. The attacks were not repeated when anticonvulsants were started.

In their study of 560 migraine patients attending a neurology clinic, Hockaday and Whitty (1969) reported alteration of consciousness during the migraine attack in 126 patients (23%). The nature of the attack was considered syncopal in 54 (10%), epileptic in 46 (8%) and was unclear in the remaining 26. These 26 included

18 cases with loss of consciousness not further detailed and eight with unusual features such as an irresistable urge to sleep, feelings of fear, or parageusia. The highest incidence of syncope was in subjects with BAM and this group, in contrast, had the lowest incidence of epileptic seizures. In a later study of BAM in children, Hockaday (1979) listed the variety of states of altered consciousness seen in 13 of 29 cases as follows: loss of consciousness, feeling of faintness, atonic drop attacks, and profound sleep from which the patient could not be fully aroused; postural syncope was also observed but no seizures with clonic movement occurred in the group.

Others have also reported a high incidence of fainting in BAM. Lapkin and Golden (1978) reviewed 30 patients with BAM followed for between 6 months and 3 years. There were 17 boys and 13 girls with age at onset ranging from 7 months to 14 years. Six patients had alteration of consciousness during attacks. In three this amounted to syncope without convulsive movement and in three others there was transient confusion. Patients were grouped according to the number of recurrent neurological symptoms referable to the basilar system: all children with loss of consciousness had at least two such symptoms present, interpreted as reflecting the severity of the underlying disturbance. Swanson and Vick (1978) reviewed 12 cases of BAM presenting to them over a 10-year period. Eight patients suffered from bouts of loss of consciousness lasting 1 to 10 min during one or more attacks. One was said to have slumped toneless. None showed convulsive movements. Whether the bouts were syncopal, secondary to hypotension, or akinetic seizures secondary to brainstem ischaemia as proposed by Bickerstaff (1961b) is uncertain. The very abrupt onset of the episodes suggested the latter in at least two cases.

The occurrence of features of epilepsy during migraine attacks

There have been many reports of epilepsy occurring during migraine attacks. Most relate to selected case material, from hospital studies, and some imply that the phenomenon is not rare in what is essentially a benign disorder. However, patients with similar features, whose migraine proves symptomatic of underlying organic disease have often, by definition, been excluded from the studies. The relative frequency with which unconsciousness and epilepsy may occur in the course of non-symptomatic migraine is therefore difficult to measure. Although many studies lack clinical detail, it does appear that while consciousness is often altered or lost during the course of migraine, incontinence and tonic or clonic movements (i.e. seizures) are uncommon. The distinction is important.

Lees and Watkins (1963) observed epilepsy during non-symptomatic migraine in only three of 354 patients: one had 'a full grand mal fit at the height of one of his attacks of migraine', and two had loss of consciousness accompanied by rigidity during some attacks. Similarly, Lance and Anthony (1966) observed only two patients with one or more major epileptic seizures as part of the attack in their prospective study of 500 cases of migraine. Both patients had focal neurological symptoms during their migraine attacks. Symptomatic migraine was excluded from this study.

The rarity of features of epilepsy during migraine and the need to regard it seriously was well demonstrated by Pearce and Foster (1965). In a group of 40 patients with migraine regarded as complicated (unusual, needing investigation) three had epileptic features during their attacks: of these one whose migraine attack culminated in major epileptic fits on four occasions and another with disorientation and then loss of consciousness proved to have a cerebral angioma.

Again, of the 15 cases with migraine and epilepsy in Barolin's (1966) series of 260 patients, five had a structural abnormality – two tumours, two arteriovenous malformations and one contusion; 'some' of these cases, it is not stated which, had their seizures towards the end of migraine attacks. There were two further patients who had seizures during migraine, in whom no underlying abnormality was found. One with childhood-onset migraine on one occasion had headache lasting 30 h, followed by coma, slowing of the EEG and then two grand mal seizures. She recovered after 'dehydrating therapy' and was then free of migraine and epilepsy during 4 years of follow-up (cerebral oedema (Fitzsimons and Wolfenden, 1985) may have played a part). The second patient had left-sided migraine and sometimes towards the end of the attack showed clonic movements of the right hand.

In a study of epilepsy in 184 migraine patients referred to a neurology department, Slatter (1968) found only 14 had epilepsy and in seven this proved to be clinically unrelated. One patient with focal epileptic attacks and migraine occurring independently had a cerebral angioma. One boy with BAM and an abnormal interictal EEG had a bout of status epilepticus. One patient had a single grand mal attack after a headache of 4 days' duration. Only in four patients did an attack of migraine occasionally culminate in a grand mal attack with no 'cause' being found; the author proposed a low convulsive threshold. There were, in addition, two patients with hemiplegic migraine who, during attacks, had involuntary movements affecting one side of the face. Landrieu et al. (1979) also reported hemiconvulsions during hemiplegic migraine in an 11-year-old boy, and Rossi et al. (1980) observed 'clonus' in two children in a series of 40 with migraine complicated by sensory and motor signs and symptoms or both.

Deonna et al. (1984) noted that four children in a series of 195 with epilepsy also had migraine. In three of these, migraine attacks were occasionally a triggering factor of the seizures; and in three a migraine type of headache was prominent in the postictal phase of seizures. The authors concluded that in these cases migraine and epilepsy were separate diseases although the symptoms could coexist. Terzano et al. (1987) found that 16 (3.6%) of 450 migraine patients also had epileptic seizures. In four the two disorders were regarded as distinct conditions, the association between them being fortuitous. In five the two types of attacks arose at about the same age and were often, if not always, closely related in time so that migraine and epilepsy appeared to play a mutually triggering role. The remaining seven patients had a more particular association with occipital seizures occurring with classical migraine attacks ('intercalated attacks', see below).

There are reports of a form of complicated migraine in children in which recurrent attacks of transient weakness of one, or other, side of the body occur – so-called alternating hemiplegia syndrome (Verret and Steele, 1971). Some reports include presentations in young children acceptable as BAM; others describe onset in early infancy sometimes with tonic, and dystonic fits: the identity of these with migraine is not established (Krägeloh and Aicardi, 1980). For a fuller discussion of this topic see Chapter 6.

The rarity of epileptic features in ordinary non-symptomatic attacks is shown in epidemiological studies. Sparks (1978) did not refer to loss of consciousness during migraine in a study by questionnaire in 423 boys and 81 girls aged 10–18 years with migraine. Moreover, Bille (1962) in his exhaustive description of the features of migraine attacks in 73 children with severe migraine, stated 'in no case were there any grounds for believing that the child had epilepsy or any cause for the symptoms other than migraine'. Congdon and Forsythe (1979) did not report any instance of convulsions during migraine attacks in their large study of 300 cases of childhood migraine, although they did note a history of epilepsy in nine children.

Conclusion

Thus, feelings of faintness are common in all forms of migraine, in severe attacks, often at the peak of the headache. Loss of consciousness, sometimes syncopal, is less common but well recognized with lost or altered consciousness prominent particularly in BAM. Migraine attacks can occasionally culminate in an epileptic attack but this is so rare that all such cases require full investigation. The possibility of an underlying structural organic lesion and hence that the migraine is symptomatic should be considered even if the epileptic attack is not apparently partial in onset. The structural abnormality most often found is an arteriovenous malformation (see Chapter 1).

Acute confusional states in migraine

Confusional states in migraine are well documented. Their distinction from dysphasic syndromes is important (Rothner *et al.*, 1982): in children severe dysphasia may easily be mistaken for confusion. TGA reported in childhood migraine (Jensen, 1980) may be similarly misinterpreted – this distinction is sometimes, however, artificial as the clinical presentations may be very similar, and often both coexist.

Confusion during migraine was well documented by Liveing in 1873. In 1970, Gascon and Barlow described four children, three boys and one girl aged 8–16, who each had a single bout of disturbed sensorium and consciousness, with agitation. A presumptive diagnosis of migraine was made on the basis of characteristic visual or sensory aura and strong family history of migraine. One boy had common migraine as he got older. The authors considered that presentation with an acute confusional state was not uncommon in their experience. However, it is difficult to achieve any perspective of prevalence from the experience of specialist centres. Thus, 34 (6.8%) of 500 patients studied by Lance and Anthony (1966) had bouts of disorientation or confusion with attacks while only one of 40 children with complicated migraine reported by Rossi *et al.* (1980) had 'a sense of confusion'. Gascon and Barlow (1970) speculated that regional cerebral oedema in a midline subcortical location might underlie the symptoms with hippocampal or reticular activating mechanisms affected. Later, however, Emery (1977) suggested that if the severe slowing in the EEG associated with confusional states in the four children he studied were due to involvement of the reticular apparatus then coma would have been more likely. He concluded the confusional state was more likely due to cortical rather than brainstem dysfunction. Ehyai and Fenichel (1978) also considered ACM more likely to be due to involvement of cerebral hemisphere than brainstem. They described five children with attacks of confusion, disorientation and agitation with a mixture of apprehension and combativeness, as brief as 10 min or as long as 20 h; in one case the attack followed angiography. In one boy the acute confusional state was preceded by monocular blindness indicating involvement of the carotid distribution and in two the EEG showed unilateral slowing. In four patients attacks were repeated. Initially the confusional states clustered and then with the passage of time were replaced by more usual forms of migraine. Emery

(1977), Ehyai and Fenichel (1978) and Tinuper *et al.* (1985) reported that ACM is sometimes aborted by a period of sleep. In two cases studied by Parrino *et al.* (1986) the authors were unable to demonstrate any physiological abnormality of sleep, suggesting functional integrity of brainstem mechanisms, and they considered that transient cortical dysfunction underlies ACM. A recent detailed study of the clinical features in 12 patients, seven aged 16 or less when seen, by the same workers (Pietrini *et al.*, 1987) describes the major symptoms as a fluctuating level of consciousness, confusion and agitation, with global or partial amnesia following the attack; in all patients but one the ACM subsided within 12 h. Ictal EEG recordings showed generalized high voltage slow wave activity, sometimes asymmetrical, and frontal intermittent rhythmic delta activity, with postictal recovery and return to normal usually within 1–2 days (occasionally a week or more). The authors discuss the distinction from acute aphasic migraine, and from migraine with TGA, and suggest that the clinical and EEG features in ACM may be the result of generalized brain dysfunction (perhaps 'spreading depression') involving particularly both temporal lobes.

Prolonged coma in migraine

Migraine can rarely cause prolonged loss of consciousness. Lee and Lance (1977) described in detail seven migraine patients (one a child) who had episodes of stupor lasting for from a few hours up to 5 days, with other neurological features suggesting disturbance of the vertebrobasilar and posterior cerebral circulation. Their case no. 2, a boy aged 17 years, had attacks repeated every 2–3 months over a 2-year period in which some hours of severe frontal headache, with vomiting, vertigo, ataxia, hyperacusis and confusion, were followed by drowsiness, then a stuporous state – in which he responded only to painful stimuli and loud noise – lasting between 3 and 18 h. He recovered fully after each attack, but was amnesic for the duration of the stupor. The authors discuss the important differential diagnosis of this presentation, which includes *inter alia* drug intoxication, vertebrobasilar insufficiency, posterior fossa tumour and porphyria. They stress the benign prognosis, with full recovery, in their cases, but cite a similar presentation with fatal outcome (Guest and Woolf, 1964). They considered that the prolonged periods of coma occurred on the basis of hypothalamic or brainstem ischaemia affecting the reticular activating system. A more recent interesting report describes a family with hemiplegic migraine studied over 40 years (Fitzsimons and Wolfenden, 1985). Coma or profound stupor often precipitated by trivial head injury were the cardinal features in the seven patients. Febrile meningoencephalitis was an associated feature in many attacks, as was the ultimate appearance of acute or chronic cerebellar ataxia. The coma was associated with cerebral oedema demonstrated by CT scanning and angiography. On occasions the oedema became severe and life-threatening and artificial ventilation became necessary. Cerebral oedema in hemiplegic migraine has been reported previously (New and Scott, 1975; Harrison, 1981) and is in keeping with Goltman's (1936) observation of migrainous cerebral oedema while performing burr hole biopsy for suspected brain tumour. The findings are again compatible with spreading depression leaving in its wake inactive and oedematous pools of neurones, as seen in animal models (Grafstein, 1956; Schadé, 1959). Intra-arterial radioisotope techniques have demonstrated how during classical migraine focal cerebral hyperaemia is followed by widespread oligaemia (Lauritzen and Olesen, 1984). This may be secondary to changes in salt and water metabolism mediated through hypothalamic abnormality (Ostfeld *et al.*, 1955; Herberg, 1975; Lauritzen and Olesen, 1984). The importance of these observations is that they describe potentially reversible phenomena which could explain how the deficit following a migraine attack usually regresses. As infarction is so rare in migraine it is likely that oedema and Leão effects contribute to the neuronal dysfunction to a greater extent than the oligaemic mechanisms emphasized previously.

Visual symptoms in migraine

In a series of 244 children attending a migraine clinic, Hachinski *et al.* (1973) found 47 boys and 53 girls whose migraine started between age 2 and 17 years (mean 8) and who reported visual symptoms, these tending to be stereotyped for each patient. Seventy-seven children had experienced visual impairment or binocular scotomata. Total obscuration of vision was more common than hemianopia and altitudinal or quadrantic defects were unusual. Scotomata were stars, squares, circles, or squiggles usually moving and evolving, occasionally fixed and unchanging, described as throbbing, spinning, flickering and swimming, and well defined or shimmering and sparkling. Many had, in addition to the binocular visual symptoms or bilateral scotomata, other symptoms suggesting brainstem as well as posterior cerebral involvement. Sixteen children had visual distortions or hallucinations or both suggesting involvement more anteriorly, of temporoparietal regions. The remaining seven children had monocular symptoms, indicating ophthalmic artery involvement; again these were either obscurations or scotomata. The paper is well illustrated with verbal and graphic detail. Plant (1986) also discusses visual phenomena of migraine very fully. In other childhood studies Bille (1962) found a higher incidence of visual aura (70%) in a selected group of children with pronounced migraine than in his overall school migraine population (50.1%). Scotoma occurred in 30% of the PMi group and scintillations in 40%. The usual duration of the visual aura varied from 1 min (two children) to about half an hour (two children) with most lasting a few or 5 min (39 children). Congdon and Forsythe (1979) described the visual auras in 94 (31%) of their series of 300 children as visual blurring (33), diplopia (14), field loss (four), 'everything goes small' (five), stars or flashes of light (17), coloured circles (9), spots (10) and 'everything goes red' (two).

In a discussion of visual symptoms in children with epilepsy, Deonna *et al.* (1984) described the visual phenomena experienced as part of their seizures by 12 of 195 epileptic children as negative (complete or partial loss of vision) in six and positive (phosphene, visual distortion) in five (six). The visual symptoms were brief, lasting only a few seconds or up to a few minutes. In 10 of the 12 cases other epileptic phenomena occurred in immediate relationship to the visual disturbance, and in the remaining two, other epileptic phenomena occurred at other times. The visual symptoms were inconstant, or only very occasional, in seven. Only three of the children could be regarded as having occipital lobe epilepsy with definite occipital spike foci (blocked by eye opening in one case) in their EEG (see below). Another four of the 195 children had migraine as well: two of them had visual disturbances during their migraine attacks, but never in association with their epilepsy.

Conclusion

Thus, it is clear that negative and positive visual phenomena occur in both migraine and epilepsy – not surprisingly with 'a common denominator' of underlying neuronal dysfunction. The duration of the symptoms and all other features of the case including EEG changes need to be considered in differentiating one from the other. The distinction may be difficult in clinical practice but clearly has important implications for therapy.

Occipital lobe epilepsy and 'intercalated migraine'

Continuous occipital or posterior temporal or parietal high voltage slow and sharp wave activity that is completely or significantly suppressed by eye opening, and augmented by hyperventilation is a well known although rare EEG abnormality in children. It has been reported as part of a syndrome of BAM with severe EEG change and infrequent generalized or focal seizures, heralded by a visual aura (Camfield et al., 1978; Panayiotopoulos, 1980). It is also well recognized in some forms of childhood epilepsy with visual aura (Gastaut, 1950, 1982; Beaumanoir, 1983; Deonna et al., 1984). Gastaut (1982, 1985) considers that epilepsy with visual symptoms, and occipital spike-wave abnormality showing attenuation on eye opening, is an identifiable syndrome: 'benign epilepsy of childhood with occipital paroxysms'. He noted that postictal headache, rarely hemicranial, occurred in 33% of 53 patients, with migraine-like nausea and vomiting in 17% and he postulated that these migrainous symptoms were the result of vascular changes which accompanied the occipital ictal activity affecting children already predisposed to migraine. It is most likely that Gastaut's cases and those described by Camfield et al. (1978) and Panayiotopoulos (1980) are the same (epileptic) syndrome, to be distinguished from BAM on the basis of the EEG abnormality.

Newton and Aicardi (1983), reporting 16 children with seizures and this EEG abnormality, did not consider that the cases formed a benign syndrome of childhood epilepsy. The aetiology of their cases was mixed and response to treatment poor in 11. Some of their cases resembled the syndrome of BAM with severe EEG change described above. Only seven of the 16 cases experienced visual symptoms. The subject is discussed further by Terzano et al. (1987), who observed seven patients with 'intercalated attacks' (sic) of occipital epilepsy with migrainous features.

Conclusion

While the *specificity* of occipital lobe epilepsy remains in doubt, the syndrome of seizures with visual symptoms, and occipital spike-and-wave abnormality showing attenuation on eye opening, is well described. Postictal headache, sometimes hemicranial and with nausea and vomiting, may occur, when the clinical picture may resemble migraine. It is most likely that the cases of so-called BAM with severe EEG abnormalities and infrequent seizures reported in the literature fall into this category of epilepsy. The reader is referred to Chapter 6 for a fuller discussion of the syndrome(s) of occipital epilepsy, and to the volume *Migraine and Epilepsy* (Andermann and Lugaresi, 1987). The distinction from BAM, in which the resting EEG is normal, and the ictal EEG shows transient posterior slow, or frontal fast, activity only (Swanson and Vick, 1978; Parain and Samson-Dollfus, 1984) is important.

Seizure headaches

This term refers to attacks where headache is the sole clinical manifestation of a seizure. Pain, both cephalic and abdominal, during epileptic seizures overt in other ways is well recognized although rare. Young and Blume (1983) observed that 24 (2.8%) of 858 epileptic patients experienced pain during their attacks – cephalic in 11 and abdominal in only three. In addition there are many reports of recurrent and periodic (*sic*) syndromes which combine, *inter alia,* nausea, vomiting, fever, vasomotor disturbance, abdominal pain and headache. Sometimes these disorders are interpreted as a form of epilepsy (O'Donohoe, 1971); this remains a difficult and controversial area. In general these symptoms should only be regarded as epileptic when the diagnosis of epilepsy stands clearly on other grounds, including alteration of consciousness, and EEG change. Similarly, recurrent visceral and vegetative symptoms of this sort are often attributed to migraine, and labelled as abdominal migraine, or equivalents of migraine, without proper evidence, and with sometimes unfortunate implications for management and outcome. These aspects are discussed in Chapter 4.

The term 'seizure headache' has been more properly used for some rather better delineated syndromes where headache with or without vomiting is the sole clinical manifestation of the attack. Millichap (1978) considered that in 19 of 100 children with recurrent headaches these were seizure equivalents, on the basis of prior history of convulsive seizures in 15, some alteration of consciousness with the headache in four, and EEG seizure discharges in all. There have been other reports of cases where headache has been accepted as the sole clinical manifestation of an epileptic attack. Swaiman and Frank (1978) described six patients whose attacks of headache were of abrupt onset, diffuse or bifrontal, usually accompanied by nausea and vomiting, and followed by lethargy or sleep. The EEG showed spikes in four, and paroxysmal slow wave discharges in two. The authors concluded the headaches were seizures because they were diffuse and responded well to anticonvulsant treatment; also there was no familial migraine. They suggested that seizure discharges in the temporal lobe, the limbic system, and other parts of the cerebral cortex could spread to the hypothalamus and through the mesencephalic nuclei into the autonomic nervous system, with resulting headache, and other autonomic symptoms such as gastrointestinal disturbance and syncope. Laplante *et al.* (1983) described headache as an epileptic manifestation in two cases, a girl of 17 and a man of 28. The headaches were described as 'swelling, fullness, pressure, heat or flash'. Depth electrode studies and behavioural recordings showed that headache was the clinical manifestation of seizures, and at temporal lobectomy (which relieved the headaches) pathology was found in both the amygdala and hippocampus. More recently Isler *et al.* (1984) reviewed the subject of *hemicrania epileptica,* finding direct evidence of homolateral, hemicranial headache with nausea and vomiting occurring in relation to unilateral neural discharge recorded by depth electrode. They observed three patients with psychomotor epilepsy in whom stimulation reproduced acute localized homolateral headache – similar to previous spontaneous headache attacks treated unsuccessfully as migraine.

The above observations appear well based, and some of the case reports are convincing, although it is of course necessary to discount 'responsiveness' to antiepileptic medication as in any way helpful in diagnosis. However, there are important clinical difficulties. Even in subjects with known epilepsy the occurrence of headaches is highly likely to be the coincidence of two common disorders. Nevertheless, there are epileptic patients, who experience headache as part of their typical attacks, who may at other times experience similar headache as an isolated symptom. In these a presumptive clinical diagnosis of seizure headache may be made. However, without the demonstration of coincident epileptic discharge on the EEG, diagnosis of a headache as a seizure can be a matter of clinical opinion only. Repeated and detailed clinical and EEG evaluations must be carried out in an attempt to reach a well-based positive or, equally important, a negative, diagnosis. Brevity of attack is not a helpful distinguishing feature favouring a diagnosis of seizure headache: in children migraine attacks are often of short duration (15 min or less). Visceral and other vegetative (autonomic) symptoms accompany both seizures and migraine, and both are, by definition, paroxysmal events. There is a danger that inappropriate – antiepileptic – drugs may be prescribed for recurrent paroxysmal headache disorders on inadequate grounds. Where there are reasonable grounds for suspicion that a headache is the clinical manifestation of a seizure, then antiepileptic medication is of course appropriate, with the usual constraints upon dosage, and with the close monitoring for unwanted effects on concentration, learning and behaviour that is so important in childhood (Hirtz and Nelson, 1985).

Conclusion

Head pain is an uncommon, but well-recognized accompaniment of epileptic attacks. Head pain as the sole clinical manifestation of an epileptic attack (so-called seizure headache) has been observed in rare instances where EEG monitoring has shown coincidence of epileptic discharge and experience of headache. Clinical diagnosis of seizure headache can only be a matter of clinical opinion, rarely justified. Use of antiepileptic medication when diagnosis is solely on clinical grounds should be cautious, and sceptical – with due recognition of possible placebo effect, and great awareness of potential adverse effects in children.

Summary

Much has been written about the relationship(s) between migraine and epilepsy. There are reports suggesting a closer than chance association between these two common disorders, but there is no clear epidemiological evidence as yet that migraine and constitutional epilepsy are genetically related. Similarly there is little evidence that frequent longstanding severe or complicated migraine leads to the appearance of (new) epilepsy or of paroxysmal EEG change in previously non-epileptic subjects, except in very rare instances.

Alteration and loss of consciousness occur not uncommonly during the course of migraine attacks, in relation to syncope, or to postulated brainstem reticular, or cerebral hemisphere, involvement; occasionally epileptic (sensory motor and reflex) symptoms occur as well. These features should always be fully investigated: while they may be the result of the effects of migraine in an otherwise normal subject, they may equally indicate one who is potentially epileptic either for genetic reasons or because of organic brain disease.

Other syndromes of migraine well recognized in childhood include acute confusional migraine and also (rarely) migraine stupor. These, together with dysphasic migraine, and migraine with transient global amnesia, may cause difficulty in diagnosis, but in retrospect, after detailed clinical appraisal and full investigation, can be recognized as non-epileptic phenomena.

In occipital epilepsy disturbances with posterior slow and sharp wave activity suppressed by eye opening, and visual symptoms, may be associated with or followed by severe headache with nausea and vomiting, when the clinical picture closely resembles migraine. It is likely that some cases reported as BAM with EEG abnormalities and seizures are examples of this form of epilepsy, in which migraine has been provoked by the seizure (intercalated migraine). There is disagreement about the nature of so-called occipital epilepsy: some have suggested that it is a specific and benign syndrome but others describe similar EEG findings with or without visual symptoms in epileptic disorders of mixed aetiology and varied outcome. Distinction of these seizure disorders from migraine is clearly of paramount importance.

Seizure headaches may also be confused with migraine and in most clinical situations the distinction cannot be made with certainty. Headache as part of a seizure is rare but well recognized (and to be separated from the extremely common phenomenon of postictal headache). There are some epileptic subjects who experience headache as part of their typical attacks who may at other times experience similar headache as an isolated symptom: a clinical diagnosis of seizure headache may be appropriate, although it is more likely that even in epileptic subjects the occurrence of isolated headache is mere coincidence. EEG demonstration of epileptic discharge at the same time as the headache is necessary for firm diagnosis, and clinical diagnosis must always be cautious.

Chapter 8

Pathophysiology and precipitants of migraine

R. C. Peatfield

Introduction

It is inevitable that very little research on the pathophysiology of migraine has been done specifically in children, although children have been the subject of a number of empirical trials of dietary manipulation in the hope of preventing attacks. Although available evidence derived from children will be emphasized in this chapter, so much of the work has been done on adults that these studies must figure largely in any comprehensive account. It is assumed, without direct evidence, that the pathophysiologies of migraine in children and in adults are not so dissimilar as to invalidate a combined approach.

There is no universally accepted integrated pathogenetic scheme for the migraine attack. As new epidemiological ideas, and in particular new techniques of investigation become available more evidence is added to the 'jig-saw', but it remains imperative to resist the temptation to provide a scheme going beyond the available evidence. Therefore, much of what follows will consist of dissociated observations offered in the hope that readers may be inspired to explore the 'gaps'.

Pathophysiology of migraine

Origin of head pain

The pain of headache is believed to originate from dilated sensitized blood vessels. It has been known for nearly two centuries that digital pressure on the superficial scalp arteries will relieve the discomfort temporarily. During headache there is an increase in the amplitude of pulsations in the superficial temporal artery, and treatment with ergotamine simultaneously reduces the pulsations and the headache (Graham and Wolff, 1938). Headache is eliminated by exposing subjects to an increased gravitational force in a centrifuge, and worsened immediately afterwards (Kunkle *et al.*, 1948). There is some evidence of increased extracranial blood flow during headache, although no change could be demonstrated in temporal muscle blood flow during unilateral common migraine attacks (Jensen and Olesen, 1985). In about one-third of cases the pain is better ameliorated by carotid occlusion in the neck than by superficial temporal artery occlusion in the forehead (Drummond and Lance, 1983) – it is thought that the pain in such patients originates in the meningeal circulation (Mayberg *et al.*, 1981). It may be possible to abort a migrainous headache completely by sustained pressure on the superficial temporal artery during the aura phase of a classical attack (Lipton, 1986).

In sequential recordings of the arterial pulsations in the superficial temporal artery (Tunis and Wolff, 1953) high amplitudes were also seen 3 days before the onset of a headache, which suggests that arteries have to be sensitized by a 'sterile inflammatory response' in order for the patients to experience the vasodilatation as headache; inflammatory mediators have been found in subcutaneous fluid taken from the scalp during an attack (Chapman et al., 1960).

The inhalation of amyl nitrite increases the intensity of non-specific 'tension type' headaches (Martin and Mathews, 1978), which suggests that they too are associated with vasodilatation. In contrast there is no convincing rise in scalp EMG activity in continuous headache of this kind (Bakal and Kaganov, 1977; Nuechterlein and Holroyd, 1980); there may be an increase during common migraine attacks, but it is never sufficient to cause ischaemic pain (Clifford et al., 1982). There is, indeed, no real evidence that these various types of idiopathic headache differ fundamentally in any way other than in degree of severity (Featherstone, 1985; Waters, 1986).

Cerebral blood flow in migraine

The most reliable studies of cerebral blood flow in migraine are those of Olesen and his colleagues in Copenhagen, who now use a tomographic apparatus to display inhaled radiolabelled xenon being washed out of the brain. They have been unable to demonstrate any change in cerebral blood flow in either induced or spontaneous common migraine attacks (Olesen et al., 1981; Lauritzen and Olesen, 1984). In classical migraine, by contrast, a wave of oligaemia can be demonstrated, most commonly moving forwards from the occipital pole (Lauritzen and Olesen, 1984; Olesen, 1985) – this corresponds to the site of the focal symptoms, but seldom if ever is flow low enough to produce any ischaemic disturbance in its own right. The oligaemia crosses the boundaries between the main cerebral arteries, but it stops at primary interlobar sulci. Sometimes there is a transient focal hyperaemia before the oligaemic phase, and headache often begins during the latter.

Spreading depression of Leão

During the aura of a typical classical migrainous attack scintillations move across the visual field at a rate corresponding to 3 mm of cortex per minute, which is similar to the rate of propagation of the 'spreading depression of Leão' first described in 1944 (Leão, 1944). Indirect evidence that this is indeed the mechanism comes not only from the similar rate of propagation of the oligaemic wave in cerebral blood flow studies, but also from experimental studies in the rat, in which similar cerebral blood flow changes can be seen to be related closely to a wave of spreading depression of electrical activity induced by directly stimulating the exposed cortex (Pearce, 1985; Lauritzen 1985, 1987). In addition, in man impaired cerebral blood flow responses to psychological activation and hyperventilation are confined to the oligaemic areas, suggesting that local rather than global factors are determining the cerebral blood flow abnormality. During migraine attacks CO_2 reactivity is decreased in the hypoperfused areas while autoregulation to blood pressure changes is preserved – a pattern opposite to that seen in cerebrovascular disease (Olesen 1985).

Gardner-Medwin (1981) has shown that hypercapnia or amyl nitrite will inhibit spreading depression in the rat, which provides an alternative explanation for the inhibition of scintillation induced by these agents, previously believed to indicate that the cortical symptoms were induced by spasm (Marcussen and Wolff, 1950; Hare, 1966).

The phenomena that may be involved as triggers of spreading depression in spontaneous migraine attacks remain obscure, as does the relationship of spreading depression to the pathogenesis of the headache (Peatfield, 1986).

Platelets and serotonin release

There is now considerable evidence that the platelet release reaction occurs in migraine. Increased platelet microaggregates are found in the circulation both during (Grotemeyer et al., 1983) and between (Hanington et al., 1981) attacks. Many groups of workers have shown increased in vitro aggregability of platelets to agents such as ADP and serotonin in blood taken during attacks, and probably also between them (see Lechner et al., 1985). Beta-thromboglobulin levels are higher at least in some patients during, and perhaps also between, migrainous attacks (Gawel et al., 1979; Lechner et al., 1985; Peatfield, 1986). It seems likely that the increased excretion of serotonin metabolites during an attack (Curran et al., 1965) is due to the liberation of serotonin bound to platelet granules, and perhaps other sites as well. Serotonin may itself enhance platelet aggregation (De Clerck and Herman, 1983). A soluble factor has been demonstrated in plasma during attacks which will liberate serotonin from platelets taken from migraine patients between attacks (Anthony et al., 1968; Mück-Seler et al., 1979) or from normal subjects (Dvilansky et al., 1976).

In addition, the active uptake of serotonin into platelets seems to be disturbed in migraine patients, at least during and immediately after an attack (e.g. Pradalier et al., 1983a). Nevertheless the absolute amount of serotonin released from platelets is small, and, in any case, much higher levels (e.g. following intravenous infusion or in the carcinoid syndrome) are not associated with headache at all (Fozard, 1982), so serotonin is unlikely to be the sole mediator of headache.

It has been suggested that generalized serotonin depletion, which might suppress the descending tracts from the midbrain raphe nuclei that are known to modulate the pain threshold, plays a role in the aetiology of migraine. However, methysergide, a drug of proven efficacy in migraine prophylaxis, is actually hyperalgesic in experimental animals (Roberts, 1984), and chronic serotonin depletion with reserpine causes migraine to disappear (Nattero et al., 1976). It seems more probable that a reduced pain threshold relates more to the pathogenesis of chronic headache than to migraine (Lancet, 1984; Peatfield, 1986).

Endogenous peptide levels

A number of workers have measured the levels of various endogenous opioids in both plasma and CSF in headache patients. CSF beta-endorphin levels were significantly reduced in 11 migraine patients, particularly in those with interparoxysmal headache (Genazzani et al., 1984). Plasma beta-endorphin levels in migraine patients between attacks seem to be normal, while studies during attacks have not yet given consistent results, with some groups reporting higher, some unchanged (perhaps using samples taken at the end of attacks), and some lower levels (Anselmi et al., 1980; Bach et al., 1985; Peatfield, 1986). Patients with chronic daily headache, however, have reduced levels in almost all the published series (Baldi *et al.*, 1982; Peatfield, 1986). It may be that the stress of a migraine attack can cause a surge of this peptide, whereas chronic daily headache leads to its depletion, but more studies need to be done.

Innervation of blood vessels

There has been a lot of recent work on the autonomic control of the cranial circulation in experimental animals. Nerve endings containing a wide variety of transmitters have been demonstrated by immunohistochemistry in both pial vessels and branches of the internal and external carotid arteries (Table 8.1). High levels of substance P have been found in cranial arteries in the cat, and these are significantly lowered by excising the trigeminal ganglion (Norregaard and Moskowitz, 1985). The opioid analgesic dynorphin B has also been found on larger cerebral arteries – this peptide does not appear to have any direct effect on vessel diameter, but it may modulate pain perception (Moskowitz *et al.*, 1986). *In vivo* studies in the monkey by Lance and his colleagues in Australia have shown that

Table 8.1 Immunohistochemistry of cranial blood vessels

Authors	Transmitter identified	Site	Possible action
Mayberg *et al.*, 1981	Serotonin	Meninges	
Griffith and Burnstock, 1983	Serotonin	Meninges	
Edvinsson *et al.*, 1980	Vasoactive intestinal peptide	Meninges	
Pipili and Poyser, 1981	Prostaglandins	Meninges	
Moskowitz, 1984	Substance P	Meninges	Dilatation Inflammation (Trigeminal; sensory)
Edvinsson, 1985 Edvinsson and Uddman, 1987	Neuropeptide Y	Pial	Constrictor (sympathetic)
Edvinsson, 1985 Edvinsson and Uddman, 1987	Vasoactive intestinal peptide	Pial	Dilatation (parasympathetic)
Gibbins *et al.*, 1984	Vasoactive intestinal peptide	Larger cerebral and extracerebral arteries	Dilatation
Edvinsson, 1985	Substance P	Larger cerebral arteries	Dilatation ? sensory role too
Edvinsson, 1985	Gastrin-releasing peptide	Larger cerebral arteries	? Sensory role
Moskowitz *et al.*, 1986	Dynorphin B	Larger cerebral arteries	Modulation of pain fibres
Jansen *et al.*, 1986	Neuropeptide Y	Temporal arteries	Potentiation of noradrenaline vasoconstriction
Jansen *et al.*, 1986	Vasoactive intestinal peptide Substance P Calcitonin gene-related peptide		Relaxation of arteries previously constricted by prostaglandin $F_{2\alpha}$

stimulation of the locus coeruleus in the brainstem produces vasoconstriction of the internal carotid artery, and vasodilatation in the external carotid circulation via the facial and from there the greater superficial petrosal nerve (Lance et al., 1983). Flushing in response to stimulation of the trigeminal nerve or ganglion is predominantly mediated as a reflex via the brainstem in both the cat (Lambert et al., 1984) and the monkey (Goadsby et al., 1986). This vasodilatation is resistant to agents blocking noradrenaline, histamine and acetylcholine receptors, but is blocked by antisera to vasoactive intestinal polypeptide (Goadsby and MacDonald, 1985).

In studies in vivo Moskowitz (1984) has shown that sensory fibres in cerebral blood vessels (for example the middle cerebral artery of the cat) enter the brain via the trigeminal nerve. There is a close relationship between trigeminal cells innervating cerebral vasculature and related parts of the dura and those innervating the skin of the forehead, which might underlie the referral of headache pain to the forehead (O'Connor and van der Kooy, 1986).

Precipitants of migraine

Stress

Many patients with recurrent migraine associate their attacks with stress – in 583 unselected clinic patients with 'severe headache' (Ziegler, 1979), 15% felt their headaches were always precipitated by emotional tension, 50% were usually so precipitated, 21% sometimes and 14% never. In an earlier survey 67% of adult migraine patients reported that headaches had been precipitated by emotional factors (Selby and Lance, 1960), and similar results were obtained, again in adults, by Henryk-Gutt and Rees (1973). In one study of children 32 out of 37 reported that attacks could be triggered by emotional upsets (Maratos and Wilkinson, 1982), while Leviton et al. (1984a) found that 33% of 11–12-year-olds related headaches to an especially hard day at school or home, and this figure rose to 65% in 17–21-year-olds. Headache was attributed to stress in 30% of 198 unselected elementary school students, and 40% of 660 secondary school students (Passchier and Orlebeke, 1985). In some patients the headache follows the stress, such as immediately after a task has been completed by a deadline. In adults headaches seem commoner on Saturdays than on any other day of the week (Barrie et al., 1968), although in children they seem commoner on weekdays and especially Fridays (Dalton and Dalton, 1979; Leviton et al., 1984b). The concept of a specific striving perfectionist personality in migraine patients, unable to express emotions openly, is no longer generally accepted (Blanchard et al., 1984). This may reflect the personalities of clinic patients who have taken the trouble to seek advice about their headaches, and not be a feature found in headache patients drawn indiscriminately from a general population (Henryk-Gutt and Rees, 1973).

There is as yet little evidence to suggest that catecholamines play any significant role in the pathogenesis of any of the phases even of a classical migraine attack (Peatfield, 1986) – the bulk of the changes that have been demonstrated seem likely to be secondary to the stress of attacks.

There are remarkably few objective psychological studies on stress levels in migraine patients that use controls and/or standardized psychological tests. Personality scale studies in small groups of self-selected patients have shown higher levels of anxiety (Harrison, 1975; Ziegler, 1979), but this seems less significant than the depression which occurs in such patients (Blumer and Heilbronn, 1982). In a comparison of 73 migraine and 73 control children, those with migraine were rated by their parents as significantly more sensitive, tidy and less physically enduring (Bille, 1962). Cunningham *et al.* (1987) showed that children with migraine scored less well than pain-free control children on rating scales for social competence, anxiety and happiness. They did not differ, however, from children with chronic musculoskeletal pain, which suggests the abnormalities are the result and not the cause of the pain.

Epidemiological evidence drawn from population surveys provides little evidence of a true distinction between migraine and tension headache, suggesting instead that many, if not all, such patients lie on a continuum (Sjaastad, 1980; Waters, 1986). Neurophysiological studies of scalp muscle activity do not show higher levels in so-called tension headache patients (Martin and Mathews, 1978; Ziegler, 1979), and many authorities now regard the term as misleading, preferring to manage all patients with attacks of headache as if they had migraine.

Stress, then, may underlie the decision a patient makes to seek medical advice about his headache, and may be closely linked to the development of attacks in a susceptible patient. Whether stress makes any contribution to the susceptibility itself is less clearly understood. There can be little doubt, however, that anxiety plays a major role in increasing the perceived severity of the headache in many patients, and that well-informed reassurance from the clinician may contribute much more to the relief obtained than drug or other therapy (Kessel, 1979) – witness the high rate of spontaneous remissions seen in many trials (e.g. Peatfield *et al.*, 1983).

Visual stimulation

Association of the onset of headaches with intense light is common in both children and adults: it was reported by 4.8% of the children experiencing headache in the epidemiological study of Passchier and Orlebeke (1985) and by 2% of another series of 300 children (Congdon and Forsythe, 1979). In a questionnaire survey 30% of 138 adult migraine patients, but only 7% of 68 muscle contraction headache patients, reported precipitation by exposure to sunlight (Vijayan *et al.*, 1980). Certain types of visual pattern can also precipitate visual discomfort or even headache (Wilkins *et al.*, 1984). Pearce (1984a) reports two patients whose headaches were precipitated by a match flame, and four by an electric light bulb – an after-image was followed within seconds by a scotoma with scintillating coloured edges. The clearly cortical nature of these stimuli suggests that these headaches (and perhaps migraine in general) are neural in origin (Pearce, 1984a). Young people, because of their attendance at discotheques, may be particularly at risk of light- or pattern-induced migraine.

Fasting and hypoglycaemia

Headache is often associated with a missed meal; this was reported in 20–25% of children seeking advice about headaches (Leviton *et al.*, 1984a), although it was less common in a study based on an appeal in the press (Dalton and Dalton, 1979). Of course it is difficult to dissociate the effects of hypoglycaemia from simultaneous stress.

Migraine is rare among diabetics (Burn *et al.*, 1984), often settling as the patients develop diabetes and recurring during spontaneous, deliberate or fasting hypoglycaemia (Blau and Pyke, 1970). However, Pearce (1971) found that migraine attacks occurred very rarely in relation to insulin-induced hypoglycaemia, and Hockaday (1975) found no instance of a migraine attack provoked by a hypoglycaemic reaction in 14 diabetic patients with migraine. Attacks may relate less to hypoglycaemia per se than to the physiological responses counteracting it (e.g. rise in free fatty acid level), which may be altered in migraine patients (Hockaday *et al.*, 1971; Hockaday, 1975).

Head injury

Generalized headache is extremely common after head injury, in both adults and children, often persisting for months or years (Cartlidge and Shaw, 1981; Lanzi *et al.*, 1985). Psychological factors are certainly important in those patients whose headaches develop long after the trauma (Cartlidge and Shaw, 1981), but there is some suggestion that early persistent headache may be associated with microscopic injury to the brain itself, to basal vascular structures or to the nerve supply to the cervical spine (Edmeads, 1985). In the Newcastle study, however, patients developing headache after discharge from hospital were significantly more likely to be depressed (Cartlidge and Shaw, 1981). Post-traumatic headaches usually settle over months; patients will benefit from reassurance that there is no major structural cause, and perhaps from antidepressant medication.

More typically migrainous attacks following immediately upon a head injury are much rarer, e.g. 37 cases among 1476 head injury patients in one series (Oka *et al.*, 1977). They have been reported in young adults (five footballers and a boxer by Matthews, 1972), but seem commoner in children (Haas and Sovner, 1969; Greenblatt, 1973; Haas *et al.*, 1975; Oka *et al.*, 1977). There is typically a lucid interval of an hour or more before the onset of focal symptoms such as hemiplegia, dysphasia, hemianopia or cortical blindness, confusion, irritability or even stupor. These symptoms can persist for several days and are sometimes, but not always, accompanied or followed by a migrainous headache. Shortlived focal seizures, which always follow the cortical deficit, have been recorded, especially in patients below the age of 8, but this does not indicate a risk of late epilepsy (Oka *et al.*, 1977). Many patients have a past or family history of migraine, and some even have relatives with similarly triggered attacks (Haas and Sovner, 1969). In the majority of cases the deficit and headache disappear without any sequelae, but some otherwise indistinguishable patients do develop brain swelling, and three fatalities have been recorded (Snoek *et al.*, 1984): unfortunately none of these came to autopsy. Several authors have speculated that mechanical stimulation of the cortex in children with malleable skulls triggers cortical spreading depression, although there is, as yet, no formal proof that this occurs (Greenblatt, 1973; Oka *et al.*, 1977; Snoek *et al.*, 1984).

Menstruation

In most large series migraine is commoner in boys than in girls before puberty. A significant proportion of adult women with migraine report that their headaches started at the menarche, especially those whose later attacks are linked to periods (Epstein *et al.*, 1975). This however was a retrospective study, and the often quoted link with menstruation is controversial. Bille (1962) observed a relationship with stage of cycle in nearly 50% of postpubertal girls, whereas Sparks (1978) found only 21% noted a relationship between attacks and cycle stage, although 73% of girls with migraine reported having their first attack between the ages of 10 and 14 years. Waters (1974a) found that while headaches may begin at menarche, the majority of girls in his study who were prepubertal were already experiencing headache. Deubner (1977) also found that menarchal status was not significantly related to the presence of headache or migraine.

The exacerbation of migraine by the contraceptive pill (Whitty *et al.*, 1966), probably with an increased risk of stroke (Bickerstaff, 1975; *Drug and Therapeutics Bulletin,* 1987), ought to be beyond the scope of most paediatricians.

Drug-induced headache

Headache, usually distinguishable from migraine, is a recognized side-effect of a wide variety of drugs, although few of these are commonly used in children. They include glyceryl trinitrate, indomethacin, dipyridamole (especially in large doses), lithium, nifedipine and ranitidine (reviewed by Peatfield, 1986). The contraceptive pill has already been mentioned.

A rebound headache is common some hours after the administration of ergotamine, particularly when it has been given repeatedly (Tfelt-Hansen and Krabbe, 1981; Saper and Jones, 1986). Such patients can rapidly become dependent on the drug, and may have to be admitted to hospital for it to be discontinued. Its half-life is so long that it is likely to accumulate if given significantly more often than monthly, and patients with more frequent attacks should instead be considered for formal prophylactic drug therapy.

Food additives

Substances specifically associated with headache include the preservative sodium nitrite, found in a variety of cured meat products (hot-dog headache) (Henderson and Raskin, 1972; Moneret-Vautrin, 1983). Headache has also been attributed to the food additives tartrazine and benzoic acid (Hanington, 1983; Royal College of Physicians, 1984), and very high doses of the sweetener aspartame (Johns, 1986). Recent studies of the well-known 'Chinese restaurant syndrome' of numbness in the neck and arms, weakness and palpitations (Raskin, 1981), suggest it may not always be due to monosodium glutamate (Ebert, 1984; Kenney, 1986).

Alcohol

Hangover should not be relevant in the majority of children, except after accidental overdoses. Although the pathogenesis remains poorly understood, it is believed that complex alcohols and other substances found in such beverages as sherry, port and red wine play a considerable role, and may provide clues to the pathogenesis of headache induced by other food substances (Peatfield, 1986).

Food intolerance

This is a contentious subject which has received much attention in recent years. There is an unfortunate tendency for favourable results in small groups of patients to be published, often with little if any rational discussion of mechanisms, and in apparent disregard of possible placebo responses. Pathogenesis, epidemiology and treatment often seem inextricably muddled, without any clear progression from laboratory science to therapeutic trials.

The recent joint report of the Royal College of Physicians and the British Nutrition Foundation (Royal College of Physicians, 1984) distinguishes:

1. *Food aversion* – avoidance of food for psychological reasons, or unpleasant bodily reactions caused by emotions associated with the food itself.
2. *Food allergy* – when there is evidence of an abnormal immunological interaction with the food.
3. The broader term *food intolerance,* which includes all reactions that are reproducible under blind conditions, whether they are mediated chemically, pharmacologically or immunologically (Pearson, 1985).

The importance of psychological responses to food was clearly demonstrated in a study in which double-blind testing could only confirm a response in four out of 23 patients considering themselves to be allergic to foods; there was clear evidence of psychiatric morbidity in the remainder (Pearson *et al.,* 1983; Rix *et al.,* 1984). The commonest psychiatric syndromes in patients with psychogenic 'pseudo food allergy' were hyperventilation and depression (Pearson, 1985). The difficulty in administering any flavoursome food item in a disguised form bedevils serious attempts to eliminate the prior conceptions of the patients; unfortunately, as Pearson (1985) remarks, much of current 'clinical ecology' rejects the principles and logic of science.

Local processes involving IgE are well established as the mechanism of allergic asthma and rhinitis (Aas and Lundkvist, 1973; Bleumink, 1983; Thompson and Bird, 1983) and of immediate urticaria induced by direct contact of antigen with the skin (Atherton, 1985). Gastrointestinal responses to ingested antigens in food such as diarrhoea, vomiting, abdominal pain and failure to thrive are common (Minford *et al.,* 1982). These are more frequent in children, probably due to the larger intake of proteins in relation to body weight and the higher intestinal permeability (Bleumink, 1983); the responses often resolve as the child grows older.

Many reactions are known to be chemically mediated, e.g. lactose intolerance in children with deficiency of its specific enzyme and lectins from a wide variety of plant foods interacting with IgE to degranulate mast cells (Helm and Froese, 1981; Moneret-Vautrin, 1983; Jones and Hunter, 1986). This group also includes headache induced by nitrites (hot-dog headache (Henderson and Raskin, 1972)) and monosodium glutamate (Kenney, 1986). Ingested substances can also cause immediate-type local responses (such as lip swelling, angio-oedema, rhinorrhoea, asthma and vomiting) within an hour of consumption, and these are soon identified by the subject or parent. These patients often show positive skin-prick test responses, and have elevated circulating IgG4 and/or IgE detected by radioimmunoassay or the radioallergosorbent test (RAST) to specific antigens (Aas and Lundkvist, 1973; Lessof *et al.,* 1980; Bleumink, 1983; Royal College of Physicians, 1984). Some of these responses, however, may again be explicable on a chemical basis; chemicals or immune reactions to food additives (preservatives, antioxidants and colourings such as tartrazine or benzoic acid (Egger *et al.,* 1983), or propionates (Werch, 1964)) have been implicated but there is as yet little direct evidence of their involvement (Royal College of Physicians, 1984).

Other subjects appear to have much more delayed responses to the foods, such as a more delayed form of asthma, eczema, abdominal pain, diarrhoea or even hyperactivity, and a wide variety of 'specific' items has been implicated, including milk, eggs and wheat. Even when blind rechallenge tests give reproducible responses, objective findings by skin-prick or positive RAST are much less consistent than in the immediate type (Lessof *et al.*, 1980; Royal College of Physicians, 1984); indeed the conclusion that food intolerance is present at all is often based only on a favourable response to a diet eliminating all but the most innocuous of foods, followed by rechallenges (Lessof *et al.*, 1980; Atherton, 1985). Commercial blood and hair tests are often fraudulent (Sethi *et al.*, 1987). Even though clinical responses often resolve with increasing age, skin tests may remain abnormal (Ford and Taylor, 1982; Bock, 1982). It seems likely that in most cases these clinical reactions are mediated by a variety of mechanisms, including direct chemical effects, while only a few are immunologically mediated. A lot of the clinical assessment and management of these patients is of doubtful veracity (David, 1985).

Atopic disorders and migraine

There have been several studies of the prevalence of atopic disorders such as asthma, eczema and hay fever among patients with migrainous headache, sometimes in comparison with patients with non-specific headache, and sometimes with historical controls (see Table 8.2 and Ziegler *et al.*, 1972). The figures have

Table 8.2 Prevalence of atopic disorders among migraine patients

Reference	Patient group	Diagnosis	Personal history of atopy (%)	Family history of atopy (%)	Both
Selby and Lance, 1960	330 Adults	Migraine	38	35	
Bille, 1962	73 Children	Migraine	24.7	31.5	
	73 Children	Controls	12.1 (n.s.)	21.9 (n.s.)	
Lance and Anthony, 1966	500 Adults	Migraine	17.4	8.2	
	100 Adults	Tension	13	6	
Waters, 1972	426 Adults	Migraine	22.1 (Eczema only)		
(population	385 Adults	Headache only	11.7	-	
survey)	486 Adults	No headache	10.3 ($P<0.05$)	-	
Medina and Diamond, 1976	376 Adults	Migraine	14.6	25.5	30.6
	Adults	Historical controls	7–10	30	
Congdon and Forsythe, 1979	300 Children	Migraine	7		

varied with the age of the subjects, but with one exception, all the studies quoted agreed in finding no excess personal or family history of atopic disorders among migraine and headache patients. Waters (1972), however, in a questionnaire survey of a community population found a significantly higher past history of eczema among subjects whose headaches were associated with two or three migraine symptoms (unilateral headache, aura or nausea) when compared with subjects with uncomplicated headaches or without any headaches.

Precipitation of headaches by specific foods

It has been known for many years that patients often report specific food items that can precipitate migraine. Although a wide variety of foods has been implicated, cheese, chocolate, citrus fruit and alcoholic drinks are most commonly mentioned by adults (Hanington, 1983). In questionnaire studies of children, cheese, chocolate and citrus fruit (Dalton and Dalton, 1979), and processed meats, chocolate, cheese and nuts (Bernstein and Del Tredici, 1983) again emerged as the foods more likely to have been consumed on the day of an attack.

The capriciousness of the phenomenon makes assessment of its prevalence in the migrainous population very difficult, and the surveys that are available are all based on the patients' responses to questioning, rather than to formal challenges. One study of the general population is that of Burr and Merrett (1983), who identified 15 subjects attributing headache to dietary factors among 475 sent a questionnaire – the proportion of the population experiencing spontaneous headaches was not recorded. Ten of these developed headaches after eating cheese and nine after chocolate; in contrast diarrhoea, vomiting and abdominal pain were attributed to foods in 51 subjects. When Paulin et al. (1985) sent a questionnaire to 1138 inhabitants of the New Zealand town of Milton, they identified 568 headache sufferers, of whom 20 blamed one or more foods, again most commonly alcohol, chocolate, coffee, cream and cheese. Among 500 food-sensitive sufferers receiving a migraine newsletter, 75% mentioned chocolate, 48% cheese, 30% citrus fruit and 25% alcoholic drinks (Hanington, 1983).

From a migraine clinic population, again of about 500 unselected patients interviewed personally (Peatfield et al., 1984), 18–19% considered themselves sensitive to cheese and/or chocolate and 11% to citrus fruit. In this study there was a highly significant correlation between these responses, so that the same patients tended to react to either all the foods or to none of them. In view of the very different biological origins of these foods this seemed to suggest that the response was biochemically rather than immunologically mediated.

In the same study 29% of the patients reported the precipitation of headaches by alcoholic drinks; again these tended to be the same subjects as those reporting dietary sensitivity (Peatfield, et al., 1984; Amery and Vandenbergh, 1987). Littlewood et al. (1988) obtained some confirmation of specific sensitivity to red wine by administering ice-cold Spanish red wine or diluted vodka through coloured straws from dark bottles: nine out of 11 patients previously associating attacks with red wine developed migrainous headaches after the wine, but none of eight taking vodka ($P < 0.001$, Fisher's exact test). All but one developed symptoms within 3 h, in contrast to the more delayed development of hangover. A similar time-course of red wine-induced headaches was reported in the cerebral blood flow studies of Olesen et al., (1981). Psychological factors, nevertheless, must be important, and Masyczek and Ough (1983) observed that headaches were more likely to develop in response to white wine if red colouring matter had been added.

Use of elimination diets in migraine patients

Pioneering attempts to use elimination diets in adult migraine patients are reviewed by Mansfield (1986); more recently Grant (1979) reported that 51 out of 60 patients became headache-free once an average of ten common foods (e.g. wheat, orange, eggs, tea, coffee, chocolate, milk and beef) had been eliminated from the diet. The patients also discontinued the contraceptive pill, alcohol and ergotamine, and avoided active and passive smoking, hunger and excessive stress. This study has been criticized on a number of grounds (Hawkins, 1979): it is difficult to establish which of a wide variety of manoeuvres was actually causing the headaches to settle, all the studies were done openly, and the end-point chosen for food rechallenge was not headache but a non-specific rise in the pulse rate. No attempt seems to have been made to eliminate the placebo effect of an enthusiastic and sympathetic clinician, nor psychological responses to certain foods. The study provides no evidence that the response (if real at all) is due to an antigen–antibody reaction of any kind.

Monro et al. (1980) reported a further study of 47 patients from the National Hospital, Queen Square, London, of whom only 33 completed open rotation and elimination diets: 23 were able to incriminate one or more specific foods, such as milk, cereal, chocolate, egg, fish, cheese, orange or rice. These authors claimed a good correlation between RAST results and responses to specific foods in individual patients. However, errors inherent in RAST binding (Merrett et al., 1980) at the low levels reported in this study are so large that these responses are well within the variability of the assay methods used. Monro et al. (1980) also attempted to use the RAST prospectively in an additional 26 patients, to predict which foods should be eliminated, but the results were no better than chance, and high total IgE levels did not appear clearly to predict responses to specific foods in this study.

In another open study all but two of 21 adult migraine subjects improved (after a 2-day exacerbation) during a week-long fast supported only by an 'elemental diet' of protein and carbohydrate hydrolysates with vitamins and minerals (Hughes et al., 1985). In subsequent rotational diets the foods said to be most likely to precipitate headaches were again chocolate, cheese, wheat and alcoholic drinks. Unfortunately, the authors did not include a control dietary period to enable them to differentiate the effects of diet from the favourable natural history of headache patients coming under intensive medical attention.

Mansfield et al. (1985) skin tested 43 adult migraine patients to a wide variety of foods: 16 had positive responses to one or more, and after these were eliminated from the diet for a month on an open basis, 11 of the 16 patients improved by more than two-thirds. In the remaining 27 patients all the skin tests were negative, and only two out of 27 improved when milk, egg, maize and wheat were eliminated from the diet. Seven of the patients with positive skin tests who improved on the elimination diet then underwent double-blind food challenge using 8 g of the suspected food in opaque white capsules: five developed an attack of migraine and all the double-blind placebo challenges were negative. It is, of course, difficult to discount the effects of suggestion in the open phase of this study, and little can be deduced about the specificity of skin tests when the patients were not challenged with any other foods.

Egger et al. (1983), working at the Hospital for Sick Children at Great Ormond Street in London, were the first to attempt a large scale double-blind trial of an elimination diet. From 99 children referred to this tertiary referral centre with 'severe frequent migraine', 88 were able to complete an 'oligoantigenic diet'. Of these 48 were atopic, which is a far higher proportion than in an age-matched migraine or control population, 41 had behaviour disturbance (mostly hyper-kinetic) even between attacks, and 14 had seizures – it is clear these patients were by no means typical of children with migraine. There was a favourable response to an open oligoantigenic diet in 82 cases, of which 74 relapsed when re-exposed on an open basis to one or more specific foods, such as milk, egg, chocolate, orange, wheat, benzoic acid or cheese. Only 40 of these 74 were able to complete the subsequent double-blind phase of the trial. In this the children were given the offending food repeatedly for at least a week, concealed in a carrot or banana rice flour base, and the response was judged positive if the child developed symptoms such as abdominal pain, distension or behavioural disorders during the next 2–7 days. Children previously responding to placebo challenges, however, had been eliminated from the study, which may have distorted the analysis. Twenty-six out of 40 children responded only when challenged by the previously identified foods, two responded only to placebo, eight to neither and four to both (P <0.001). Nevertheless, all 40 children were not challenged with all the foods; the challenges were not all carried out under medical supervision, and not all of the 40 subjects actually developed a headache after they had been challenged. The responses took an average of 2 days (range 1 hour to 7 days) to develop, which contrasts with the production of headache in sensitive adults within a matter of hours of single exposures to cheese, chocolate or red wine, and they shed little light on the mechanisms of this latter phenomenon. Many of the foods found to be active in this study are already known to contain vasoactive substances, such as amines, in any case. Serum IgE levels were not helpful in Egger's study, and certainly this work provides no evidence the mechanism is immunological in origin.

In their earlier paper Monro et al. (1980) had claimed that oral sodium cromoglycate exerted a protective effect during dietary rechallenges. The same group carried out a further double-blind study (Monro et al., 1984) of only nine patients with severe migraine, in whom the symptoms produced in rechallenge tests were largely intestinal rather than overtly migrainous (Pearce 1984b). Five of eight subjects claimed complete, and three partial, protection by oral sodium cromoglycate, and IgE complexes appeared in the serum after food challenges preceded by placebo but not after those preceded by sodium cromoglycate. The small size of this study, and the uncertainties surrounding the mode of action of sodium cromoglycate (Church and Warner, 1985) make it difficult to endorse the authors' view that it offers evidence that the drug blocks an immunological trigger in the gut wall, and the predominantly local symptoms produced by the foods in the study tell us little or nothing about triggers for migraine.

Bentley et al. (1984) studied 12 children aged 5–15 years with recurrent abdominal pain and a family history of classical migraine. Ten of the 12 improved on an open diet excluding egg, dairy produce and chocolate, but in none of the patients was the total or specific IgE (RAST) helpful in defining the causative food allergen. Three of the four children with raised IgE levels were known to be atopic.

In unselected patients Medina and Diamond (1978) did not seem to be able to alter the overall frequency or severity of migraine by diets high and low in cheese, chocolate, alcohol and related foods, but they did find that some attacks were time locked to these foods which would cause them to take place earlier. Unge et al. (1983) reported remissions in nine out of ten patients put on a vegetarian diet, attributing the response to a reduced tryptophan load. Salfield et al. (1987) completed an open comparison of a high fibre diet eliminating cheese, chocolate and citrus fruit with a control diet merely rich in fibre, in 39 unselected children with migraine. Thirty-four (87%) of the children showed at least a 20% reduction in the number of attacks during the study, which the authors attributed to reassurance given in the clinic and to more regular meals, but there was no significant difference between the effects of the two diets.

Less favourable experience with elimination diets has recently been reported by MacDonald *et al.* (1987): of 52 children studied only seven were shown to have food intolerance and 13 obtained no benefit from a 3-week elimination diet. The results in the remainder were inconclusive because of the high cost of the diet and poor compliance, spontaneous remissions or unpredictable responses on rechallenge. These authors re-emphasized the difficulties involved in the therapeutic use of diets of this kind. Moreover, strict diets are not always without hazard – a case of scurvy has been reported (Hughes *et al.*, 1986).

Laboratory investigations of these patients

From the epidemiological and clinical studies outlined it is clear that in some patients, both adults and children, attacks (although not always of headache) can be precipitated by specific foods or eliminated by manipulating the diet. From large-scale studies of relatively unselected patients it seems that only a minority of patients respond in this way, and even these do not do so consistently. Despite claims made in published trials, symptomatic responses provide few direct clues about the mechanisms involved, and laboratory studies are necessary.

Several independent studies have failed to find elevated serum IgE (Medina and Diamond, 1976; Monro *et al.*, 1980; Egger *et al.*, 1983; Merrett *et al.*, 1983; Pradalier *et al.*, 1983b) or IgG4 (Merrett *et al.*, 1983) either in migraine patients as a whole or specifically in patients giving a history of food-precipitated headaches. High levels are usually found in the minority of subjects who are atopic (Pradalier *et al.*, 1983b; Bentley *et al.*, 1984). Specific food-directed IgE levels, as measured by the RAST, were no higher in dietary adults (Merrett *et al.*, 1983) or children (Bentley *et al.*, 1984; A. V. Katchburian *et al.*, 1986, personal communication). Patients did not respond to challenges with foods to which RASTs were positive (Pradalier *et al.*, 1983b). Studies alleging otherwise are seriously flawed (Merrett *et al.*, 1980).

Investigations of complement activation in migraine during attacks have provided conflicting results. Reduced levels of the complement components C4 and C5 have been found during the prodromal phases of common but not classical migraine (Lord and Duckworth, 1978), and the same study found circulating immune complexes (by the precipitation of radiolabelled C1q) at the onset of some migraine attacks. These authors were unable to suggest a reason for the differences between common and classical attacks. Sovak *et al.* (1980) found no differences in C1 inhibitor levels between migraine subjects and controls, and Moore *et al.* (1980) found no changes in circulating complement, immunoglobulin or immune complex levels in paired samples taken during and between migraine attacks, either classical or common. All values fell within the normal range. Jerzmanowski and Klimek (1983), however, found normal C4 levels but a reduction in C3, which led them to suggest activation of the alternative pathway of the complement system. Visintini *et al.* (1986) included 46 patients with common or classical migraine (of whom two were milk sensitive) in a comparison with cluster headache – there were no differences in the concentrations of immunoglobulins, serum complement components C1q, C3, C4 or factor B, or IgG or IgM immune complexes between any of the patients and control subjects, both during and between migraine attacks. Thonnard-Neumann and Neckers (1981) found significantly fewer circulating T-lymphocytes and basophils in migraine patients, but only during attacks. The significance of these various observations is not known.

Chemical hypotheses

The finding that patients with dietary migraine are usually sensitive to chocolate, cheese and citrus fruit, rather than to only one of them suggests that they exert their effects by a common pathogenetic mechanism; antigenic similarities between these different foods seem less likely than some common chemical constituent (Glover *et al.*, 1983; Moneret-Vautrin, 1983; Peatfield *et al.*, 1984).

The first such substance suggested was tyramine, which is produced by the breakdown of protein, e.g. in cheese and game. Hanington (1967, 1983) was the first to notice the overlap between the foods often causing migraine and those (e.g. cheese, yeast extracts, pickled herring, broad bean pods and certain wines) that had been found to produce hypertensive reactions in subjects taking monoamine oxidase (MAO) inhibitors. There was already good evidence that tyramine, a substrate for MAO, is the major responsible constituent common to these foods (Blackwell *et al.*, 1967; Blackwell, 1981). Hanington carried out a placebo controlled study of the effects of oral tyramine (125 mg) in 50 patients with dietary migraine, finding that tyramine was followed by headache significantly more often than was placebo.

Since then there have been a number of similar studies, usually in small numbers, using both unselected, and dietary, migraine subjects. Forsythe and Redmond (1974) observed in 38 unselected children with migraine that headache was 'provoked' more often by placebo than by tyramine. Other studies in adults comparing tyramine with placebo have also failed to show a significant headache-inducing effect of tyramine in either dietary migraine (Moffett *et al.*, 1972; Ryan, 1974; Shaw *et al.*, 1978) or in unselected migraine patients (Ryan, 1974; Ziegler and Stewart, 1977; Boisen *et al.*, 1978). Some authors (Ghose *et al.*, 1977; Boisen *et al.*, 1978) were unable to relate tyramine-induced headache to a prior dietary history.

Chocolate contains little tyramine, and it is now believed to contain only insignificant amounts of beta-phenylethylamine, another amine reported to precipitate headache (Sandler *et al.*, 1974); more complex phenolic molecules may be much more important. Although Hanington (1974, 1983) found that chocolate from which all amines had been removed did not induce attacks in six previously susceptible subjects, Moffett *et al.* (1974) could not confirm this. They administered 44 g of commercial chocolate and matching placebo to 25 subjects complaining of chocolate-sensitive migraine, and found that eight responded only to the chocolate and five only to the placebo. Moreover, when the study was repeated in 15 of the subjects, results were reproducible in only five.

A variety of phenolic amines are found in citrus fruits, and such compounds can be detected in urine after the consumption of oranges, mustard, coffee and vanilla (Perry *et al.*, 1965). No challenge studies with these substances have been reported in migraine patients.

The explanation for the inconsistent results in some of the clinical challenge tests with crude food items, or purified constituents, may lie in the accuracy of the patient's account of precipitating factors, the timing of the challenge in relation to the last headache, and the precise nature of the responsible food (Forsythe and Redmond, 1974; Hanington, 1974). In the studies with tyramine, for example, there are wide variations in the number of headaches induced by placebo (Kohlenberg, 1982). Different patient expectations may have resulted from the administration of tyramine at home (Hanington, 1983) or in hospital (e.g. Moffett *et al.*, 1972; Kohlenberg, 1982). Reproducibility of the response has been far from perfect. In Ryan's study with tyramine (1974) only 15 out of 27 positive responders reacted again on rechallenge, and the results of Moffett *et al.* (1974) were similar. It seems likely from studies of platelet enzymes (see below) that phenolic compounds other than tyramine may be much more important.

At present all that can be said with certainty is that headaches can be precipitated by *some* substances found in food on *some* occasions in *some* patients (Kohlenberg, 1982).

Metabolism of potential mediators of dietary migraine

If phenols and/or amines are responsible it should be possible to identify one or more easily definable biochemical abnormalities in the dietary-sensitive patients, although clearly these abnormalities must be distinguished from those in the 'final common pathway' in all migraine patients whether the headaches can be precipitated by foods or not. The lack of a clearcut inheritance pattern in migraine (Lucas, 1977) does imply that there is likely to be more than one biochemical defect.

There are two major pathways for the metabolism of these substances in man: oxidation by MAO, and sulphation to water-soluble conjugates. Although oxidation is the more important pathway, up to 50% of a tyramine load may be sulphated (Smith *et al.*, 1971). Youdim *et al.* (1971) reported a reduced urinary output of sulphated tyramine metabolites in subjects with food sensitive migraine.

Enzymes for both oxidation and sulphation can be identified in the platelet, and are therefore readily available for testing in affected patients. While low levels of platelet MAO have been found in migraine patients both during (Sandler *et al.*, 1970; Bussone *et al.*, 1977; Glover *et al.*, 1977) and between (Sicuteri *et al.*, 1972; Glover *et al.*, 1981) attacks, more recent studies (Glover *et al.*, 1981) have failed to find lower values in patients with diet-precipitated headache. In contrast, the enzyme phenolsulphotransferase (PST) has been found to be lower in the platelets of these patients by two independent groups (Littlewood *et al.*, 1982; Soliman *et al.*, 1987), but in the studies to date this has only been significant for the subtype of the enzyme that sulphates pure phenols rather than tyramine. As yet the relevant substrates for this enzyme have not been discovered, although the phenolic flavonoids found in red wine are plausible candidates, and there is recent evidence that PST may be responsible for the conjugation of tyrosine residues (Roth, 1986). In addition red wine, and a number of phenols found in food and a variety of food additives, have been found to be inhibitors of the enzyme (Littlewood *et al.*, 1987), and their absorption may thereby be enhanced. It is also possible that there are deficiencies of the enzyme subtypes normally present in the gut wall.

Conclusions

Our understanding of the pathogenesis of migraine is at best fragmentary. The headache phase appears to be associated with painful vasodilatation in the scalp and/or meninges, and there is indirect evidence that the aura phase of classical attacks is related to cortical spreading depression – so far the triggers for each and the relationship between them are poorly understood. During attacks there are disturbances of cerebral blood flow, of platelet function and of endogenous opioid substances that have yet to be convincingly linked into a pathogenetic scheme, and the role of neuropeptides remains incompletely explored.

Headaches can be precipitated by stress, visual stimulation and head injury, but the mechanisms of these remain uncertain. A number of drugs and food additives will also cause headaches.

There is little doubt that migraines can sometimes be precipitated by food items, particularly cheese, chocolate, citrus fruit and some, if not all, alcoholic drinks. There are widely differing attitudes and opinions about the prevalence of dietary migraine, and its importance in the treatment of patients, both selected or otherwise, remains at best uncertain. There is virtually no evidence that the phenomenon is mediated by a classical antigen–antibody reaction to the food. Although there are many similarities to hypertensive reactions occurring in patients taking MAO inhibitors, and levels of this enzyme in the platelets are low in migraine patients, there is no evidence the enzyme is any lower in the platelets of patients with food-precipitated attacks. Two independent laboratories, however, have now found a defect of sulphation in the platelets of dietary migraine patients, and more recent studies suggest that substances found in the foods most commonly implicated inhibit this enzyme as well as being potential substrates for it. Our understanding of the later stages of the pharmacological pathway remain even less well understood.

Acknowledgements

I am grateful to a number of colleagues for their comments on this chapter, especially Vivette Glover, Anita Macdonald and Keith Rix. The text and references have been typed by Mrs Anne Drake.

References

AAS, K. and LUNDKVIST, U. (1973) The radioallergosorbent test with a purified allergen from codfish. *Clinical Allergy,* **3,** 255–261

ABROMS, I. F., YESSAYAN, L., SHILLITO, J and BARLOW C. F. (1971) Spontaneous intracerebral haemorrhage in patients suspected of multiple sclerosis. *Journal of Neurology, Neurosurgery and Psychiatry,* **34,** 157–162

AD HOC COMMITTEE (1962) Classification of headache. *Journal of the American Medical Association,* **179,** 717–718

ADAMS, R. D. and LYON, G. (1982) *Neurology of Hereditary Metabolic Diseases in Children.* Mcgraw-Hill, Hemisphere, Maidenhead

ALVAREZ, W.C. (1947) The migrainous personality and constitution: the essential features of the disease: a study of 500 cases. *American Journal of Medical Science,* **213,** 1–8

AMERY, W. K. (1983) Flunarizine, a calcium channel blocker: a new prophylactic drug in migraine. *Headache,* **23,** 70–74

AMERY, W. K. and VANDENBERGH, V. (1987) What can precipitating factors teach us about the pathogenesis of migraine? *Headache,* **27,** 146–150

AMERY, W. K., WAELKENS, J. and CAERS, I. (1986) Dopaminergic mechanisms in premonitory phenomena. In *The Prelude to the Migraine Attack* (eds W. A. Amery and A. Wauquier), Baillière Tindall, London, pp. 64–77

AMERY, W. K. and WAUQUIER, A. (eds) (1986) *The Prelude to the Migraine Attack,* Baillière Tindall London

ANDERMANN, E. and ANDERMANN, F. (1987) Migraine–epilepsy relationships: epidemiological and genetic aspects. In *Migraine and Epilepsy* (eds F. Andermann and E. Lugaresi), Butterworths, London, Chap. 19, pp. 281–291

ANDERMANN, F. and LUGARESI, E. (eds) (1987) *Migraine and Epilepsy,* Butterworths, London

ANDERSON, J. A. D., BASKER, M. A. and DALTON, R. (1975) Migraine and hypnotherapy. *International Journal of Clinical and Experimental Hypnosis,* **23,** 40–58

ANSELMI, B., BALDI, E., CASACCI, F. and SALMON, S. (1980) Endogenous opioids in cerebrospinal fluid and blood in idiopathic headache sufferers. *Headache,* **20,** 294–299

ANTHONY, M. (1983) Drugs in migraine. *Current Therapeutics,* **24,** 89–113

ANTHONY, M., HINTERBERGER, H. and LANCE, J. W. (1968) Studies of serotonin metabolism in migraine. *Proceedings of the Australian Association of Neurologists,* **5,** 109–112

APLEY, J. and HALE, B. (1973) Children with recurrent abdominal pain: how do they grow up? *British Medical Journal,* **3,** 7–9

ASHWORTH, B. (1985) Migraine, head trauma and sport. *Scottish Medical Journal,* **30,** 240–242

ATHERTON, D. J. (1985) Skin disorders and food allergy. *Journal of the Royal Society of Medicine,* Suppl. 5, **78,** 7–10

BACH, F. W., JENSEN, K., BLEGVAD, N., FENGER, M. *et al.* (1985) β-endorphin and ACTH in plasma during attacks of common and classic migraine. *Cephalalgia,* **5,** 177–182

BAIER, W. K. (1985) Genetics of migraine and migraine accompagnée: a study of 81 children and their families. *Neuropediatrics,* **16,** 84–91

BAIER, W. K. and DOOSE, H. (1985) Petit mal absences of childhood onset: familial prevalences of migraine and seizures. *Neuropediatrics,* **16,** 80–83

BAIER, W. K. and DOOSE, H. (1987) Migraine and petit mal absence: familial prevalence of migraine and siezures In *Migraine and Epilepsy* (eds F. Andermann and E. Lugaresi), Butterworths, London, pp. 293–311

BAILEY, T. D., O'CONNOR, P. S. TREDICI, T. J. and SHACKLETT, D. E. (1984) Ophthalmoplegic migraine. *Journal of Clinical Neuro-Ophthalmology,* **4,** 225–228

BAKAL, D. A. and KAGANOV, J. A. (1977) Muscle contraction and migraine headache: psychophysiologic comparison. *Headache,* **17,** 208–215

BALDI, E., SALMON, S., ANSELMI, B., SPILLANTINI, M. G. *et al.* (1982) Intermittent hypoendorphinaemia in migraine attack. *Cephalalgia,* **2,** 77–81

BARABAS, G., FERRARI, M. and MATTHEWS, W. S. (1983a) Childhood migraine and somnambulism. *Neurology,* **33,** 948–949

BARABAS, G., MATTHEWS, W. S. and FERRARI, M. (1983b) Childhood migraine and motion sickness. *Pediatrics,* **72,** 188–190

BARABAS, G., MATTHEWS, W. S. and FERRARI, M. (1984) Tourette's syndrome and migraine. *Archives of Neurology,* **41,** 871–872

BARLOW, C. F. (1984) *Headaches and Migraine in Childhood. Clinics in Developmental Medicine,* no. 91, Spastics International Medical Publications, Blackwell Scientific, Oxford

BAROLIN, G. S. (1966) Migraines and epilepsies – a relationship? *Epilepsia,* **7,** 53–66

BAROLIN, G. S. and SPERLICH, D. (1969) Migraine families – contribution to the genetic aspect. *Fortschritte Der Neurologie, Psychiatrie Und Ihrer Grenzgebiete (Stuttgart),* **37,** 521–544

BARRIE, M. A., FOX, W. R., WEATHERALL, M. and WILKINSON, M. I. P. (1968) Analysis of symptoms of patients with headaches and their response to treatment with ergot derivatives. *Quarterly Journal of Medicine,* **37,** 319–336

BASSER, L. S. (1964) Benign paroxysmal vertigo of childhood (a variety of vestibular neuronitis). *Brain,* **87,** 141–152

BASSER, L. S. (1969) The relation of migraine and epilepsy. *Brain,* **92,** 285–300

BATTISTELLA, P. A., MATTESI, P., CASARA, G. L. *et al.* (1987) Bilateral cerebral occipital calcifications and migraine-like headache. *Cephalalgia,* **7,** 125–129

BEAUMANOIR, A. (1983) Infantile epilepsy with occipital focus and good prognosis. *European Neurologie,* **22,** 43–52

BEDDOE, G. M. (1977) Vertigo in childhood. *Otolaryngologic Clinics of North America,* **10,** 139–144

BEHRENS, M. M. (1978) Headaches associated with disorders of the eye. *Medical Clinics of North America,* **62,** 507–521

BELFER, M. L. and KABAN, L. B. (1982) Temporomandibular joint dysfunction with facial pain in children. *Pediatrics,* **69,** 564–567

BENTLEY, D., KATCHBURIAN, A. and BROSTOFF, J. (1984) Abdominal migraine and food sensitivity in children. *Clinical Allergy,* **14,** 499–500

BERGER, H. G., HONIG, P. J. and LIEBMAN, R. (1977) Recurrent abdominal pain. *American Journal of Diseases in Children,* **131,** 1340–1344

BERNSTEIN, A. L. and DEL TREDICI, A. M. (1983) Migraine in children – a report of a dietary study. *Headache,* **23,** 142 (abstract)

BICKERSTAFF, E. R. (1961a) Basilar artery migraine. *Lancet,* **i,** 15–17

BICKERSTAFF, E. R. (1961b) Impairment of consciousness in migraine. *Lancet,* **ii,** 1057–1059

BICKERSTAFF, E. R. (1962) The basilar artery and the migraine – epilepsy syndrome. *Proceedings of the Royal Society of Medicine,* **55,** 167–169

BICKERSTAFF, E. R. (1964a) Aetiology of acute hemiplegia in childhood. *British Medical Journal,* **2,** 82–87

BICKERSTAFF, E. R. (1964b) Ophthalmoplegic migraine. *Revue neurologique,* **110,** 582–588

BICKERSTAFF, E. R. (1975) *Neurological Complications of Oral Contraceptives,* Clarendon, Oxford

BICKERSTAFF, E. R. (1986) Basilar artery migraine. In *Headache* (eds P. J. Vinken, G. W. Bruyn, H. L. Klawans and F. C. Rose), *Handbook of Clinical Neurology,* **48,** chap. 10, 135–140, Elsevier, Amsterdam

BILLE, B. (1962) Migraine in schoolchildren. *Acta Paediatrica,* Suppl. 136, **51,** 1–151

BILLE, B. (1973) The prognosis of migraine in schoolchildren. *Acta Paediatrica Scandinavica Supplement*, **236**, 38

BILLE, B. (1981) Migraine in childhood and its prognosis. *Cephalalgia*, **1**, 71–75

BILLE, B. (1982) Migraine in childhood. *Panminerva Medica (Torino)*, **24**, 57–62

BILLE, B., LUDVIGSSON, J. and SANNER, G. (1977) Prophylaxis of migraine in children. *Headache*, **17**, 61–63

BIRT, D. (1978) Headaches and head pains associated with diseases of the ear, nose and throat. *Medical Clinics of North America*, **62**, 523–531

BLACKWELL, B. (1981) Adverse effects of antidepressant drugs. Part 1: Monoamine oxidase inhibitors and tricyclics. *Drugs*, **21**, 201–219

BLACKWELL, B., MARLEY, E., PRICE, J. and TAYLOR, D. (1967) Hypertensive interactions between monoamine oxidase inhibitors and foodstuffs. *British Journal of Psychiatry*, **113**, 349–364

BLANCHARD, E. B., ANDRASIK, F. and ARENA, J. G. (1984) Personality and chronic headache. *Progress in Experimental Personality Research*, **13**, 303–364

BLAU, J. N. (1980) Migraine prodromes separated from the aura: complete migraine. *British Medical Journal*, **281**, 658–660

BLAU, J. N. (1986) Clinical characteristics of premonitory symptoms in migraine. In *The Prelude to the Migraine Attack* (eds W. A. Amery and A. Wauquier), Baillière Tindall, London, pp. 39–43

BLAU, J. N. (1987) Loss of migraine: when, why, and how. *Journal of the Royal College of Physicians of London*, **21**, 140–142

BLAU, J. N. and PYKE, D. A. (1970) Effect of diabetes on migraine. *Lancet*, **ii**, 241–243

BLAU, J. N. and WHITTY, C. W. M. (1955) Familial hemiplegic migraine. *Lancet*, **ii**, 115–116

BLAYNEY, A. W. and COLMAN, B. H. (1984) Dizziness in childhood. *Clinical Otolaryngology*, **9**, 77–85

BLEUMINK, E. (1983) Immunological aspects of food allergy. *Proceedings of the Nutrition Society*, **42**, 219–231

BLUMER, D. and HEILBRONN, M. (1982) Chronic muscle contraction headache and the pain-prone disorder. *Headache*, **22**, 180–183

BOCK, S. A. (1982) The natural history of food sensitivity. *Journal of Allergy and Clinical Immunology*, **69**, 173–177

BODIAN, M. (1964) Transient loss of vision following head trauma. *New York State Journal of Medicine*, **64**, 916–920

BOISEN, E., DETH, S., HÜBBE, P. *et al.* (1978) Clonidine in the prophylaxis of migraine. *Acta Neurologica Scandinavica*, **58**, 288–295

BOUSSER, M. G., CHIRAS, J., BORIES, J. and CASTAIGNE, P. (1985) Cerebal venous thrombosis. A review of 38 cases. *Stroke*, **16**, 199–213

BRADSHAW, P. and PARSONS, M. (1965) Hemiplegic migraine, a clinical study. *Quarterly Journal of Medicine (New series)*, **34**, 65–85

BRAY, P. F., HERBST, J. J., JOHNSON, D. G. *et al.* (1977) Childhood gastro-oesophageal reflux. Neurologic and psychiatric syndromes mimicked. *Journal of the American Medical Association*, **237**, 1342–1345

BREWIS, M., POSKANZER, D. C. ROLLAND, C. *et al.* (1966) Neurological disease in an English city. *Acta Neurologica Scandinavica*, **42**, suppl. 24, 1–89

BRINCIOTTI, M., GUIDETTI, V., MATRICARDI, M. and CORTESI, F. (1986) Responsiveness of the visual system in childhood migraine studied by means of VEPs. *Cephalalgia*, **6**, 183–185

BROTT, T. and LEVITON, A. (1976) Headache rounds: violence. *Headache*, **16**, 203–209

BROWN, J. K. (1977) Migraine and migraine equivalents in children. *Developmental Medicine and Child Neurology*, **19**, 683–692

BRUCE, D. A. (1984) Leading article. Delayed deterioration of consciousness after trivial head injury in childhood. *British Medical Journal*, **289**, 715–716

BRUYN, G. W. (1986) Migraine equivalents. In *Headache* (eds P. J. Vinken, G. W. Bruyn, H. L. Klawans and F. L. Rose), *Handbook of Clinical Neurology*, **48**, chap. 12, 155–171, Elsevier, Amsterdam

BURKE, E. C. and PETERS, G. A. (1956) Migraine in childhood. A preliminary report. *American Journal of Diseases of Children*, **92**, 330–336

BURN, W. K., MACHIN, D. and WATERS, W. E. (1984) Prevalence of migraine in patients with diabetes. *British Medical Journal*, **289**, 1579–1580

BURR, M. L. and MERRETT, T. G. (1983) Food intolerance: a community survey. *British Journal of Nutrition*, **49**, 217–219

BUSSONE, G., GIOVANNINI, P., BOIARDI, A. and BOERI, R. (1977) A study of the activity of platelet monoamine oxidase in patients with migraine headaches or with 'cluster headaches'. *European Neurology*, **15**, 157–162

Butterworths Medical Dictionary (2nd edn) (1978) Butterworth, London

CAERS, L. I., DE BEUKALAAR, F. and AMERY, W. L. (1987) Flunarizine, a calcium-entry blocker in childhood migraine, epilepsy and alternating hemiplegia. *Clinical Neuropharmacology*, **10**, 162–168

CAIRO, M. S., LAZARUS, K., GILMORE, R. L. and BAEHNER, R. L. (1980) Intracranial hemorrhage and focal seizures secondary to use of L-asparaginase during induction therapy of acute lymphocytic leukemia. *Journal of Paediatrics*, **97**, 829–833

CAMFIELD, P. R., METRAKOS, K. and ANDERMANN, F. (1978) Basilar migraine, seizures and severe epileptiform EEG abnormalities. *Neurology*, **28**, 584–588

CARSTAIRS, L. S. (1958) Headache and gastric emptying time. *Proceedings of the Royal Society of Medicine*, **51**, 790–791

CARTLIDGE, N. E. F. and SHAW, D. A. (1981) *Head Injury. Major Problems in Neurology Series*, W. B. Saunders, London

CASAER, P. (1987) Flunarizine in alternating hemiplegia of childhood. An International study in 12 children. *Neuropediatrics*, **18**, 191–195

CASAER, P. and AZOU, M. (1984) Letter. Flunarizine in alternating hemiplegia in childhood. *Lancet*, **ii**, 579

CASTEELS-VAN DAELE, M. (1979) Letter. Benign paroxysmal torticollis in infancy. *Acta Paediatrica Scandinavica*, **68**, 911–912

CASTEELS-VAN DAELE, M. (1982) Letter. Benign paroxysmal torticollis in infancy. *Archives of Disease in Childhood*, **57**, 638

CASTEELS-VAN DAELE, M., JAEKEN, J., VAN DER SCHUEREN, P. *et al.* (1970) Dystonic reactions in children caused by metoclopramide. *Archives of Disease in Childhood*, **45**, 130–133

CASTEELS-VAN DAELE, M., STANDAERT, L., BOEL, M., *et al.* (1981) Letter. Basilar migraine and viral meningitis. *Lancet*, **i**, 1366

CHAPMAN, L. F., RAMOS, A. O., GOODELL, H., *et al.* (1960) A humoral agent implicated in vascular headache of the migraine type. *Archives of Neurology*, **3**, 223–229

CHENG, X-M., ZIEGLER, D. K., LI, S-C., *et al.* (1986) A prevalence survey of 'incapacitating headache' in the People's Republic of China. *Neurology*, **36**, 831–834

CHRISTENSEN, M. F. and MORTENSEN, O. (1975) Long term prognosis in children with recurrent abdominal pain. *Archives of Disease in Childhood*, **50**, 110–114

CHURCH, M. K. and WARNER, J. O. (1985) Sodium cromoglycate and related drugs. *Clinical Allergy*, **15**, 311–320

CHUTORIAN, A. M. (1974) Abstract. Benign paroxysmal torticollis, tortipelvis and retrocollis in infancy. *Neurology*, **24**, 366–367

CLARKSON, P. M., GOMEZ, M. R., WALLACE, R. B. and WEIDMAN, W. H. (1967) Central nervous system complications following Blalock–Taussig operation. *Pediatrics*, **39**, 18–23

CLIFFORD, T., LAURITZEN, M., BAKKE, M. *et al.* (1982) Electromyography of pericranial muscles during treatment of spontaneous common migraine attacks. *Pain*, **14**, 137–147

COHEN, R. J. and TAYLOR, J. R. (1979) Persistent neurologic sequelae of migraine: a case report. *Neurology*, **29**, 1175–1177

COLLIN, C., HOCKADAY, J. M. and WATERS, W. E. (1985) Headache and school absence. *Archives of Disease in Childhood*, **60**, 245–247

COMMISSION ON CLASSIFICATION AND TERMINOLOGY (1981) International League against Epilepsy: proposed revisions of clinical and EEG classification of epileptic seizures 1981. *Epilepsia*, **22**, 489–501

CONGDON, P. J. and FORSYTHE, W. I. (1979) Migraine in childhood: a study of 300 children. *Developmental Medicine and Child Neurology*, **21**, 209–216

CONNOR, R. C. R. (1962) Complicated migraine: a study of permanent neurologic and visual defects caused by migraine. *Lancet*, **ii**, 1072–1075

COULTHARD, M. (1984) Recurrent abdominal pain: a psychogenic disorder? *Archives of Disease in Childhood*, **59**, 189–190

CROWELL, F. G., STUMP, D. A., BILLER, J. *et al.* (1984) The transient global amnesia–migraine connection. *Archives of Neurology*, **41**, 75–79

CUNNINGHAM, S. J., McGRATH, P. J., FERGUSON, H. B. *et al.* (1987) Personality and behavioural characteristics in pediatric migraine. *Headache,* **27,** 16–20

CURRAN, D. A., HINTERBERGER, H. and LANCE, J. W. (1965) Total plasma serotonin, 5-hydroxyindoleacetic acid and *p*-hydroxy-*m*-methoxymandelic acid excretion in normal and migrainous subjects. *Brain,* **88,** 997–1010

CURTIS-BROWN, R. (1925) A protein poison theory. *British Medical Journal,* **1,** 155–156

DALESSIO, D. J. (ed.) (1987a) *Wolff's Headache and other Head Pain,* 5th edn, Oxford University Press, Oxford

DALESSIO, D. J. (ed.) (1987b) Toxic vascular headache. In *Wolff's Headache and Other Head Pain,* 5th edn, Oxford University Press, Oxford, pp. 136–171

DALSGAARD-NIELSEN, T., ENGBERG-PEDERSEN, H. and HOLM, H. E. (1970) Clinical and statistical investigations of the epidemiology of migraine. *Danish Medical Bulletin,* **17,** 138–148

DALTON, K. and DALTON, M. (1979) Food intake before migraine attacks in children. *Journal of the Royal College of General Practitioners,* **29,** 662–665

DAVID, T. J. (1985) The overworked or fraudulent diagnosis of food allergy and food intolerance in children. *Journal of the Royal Society of Medicine,* Suppl. 5, **78,** 21–31

DAVID, T. J. (1987) Reactions to dietary tartrazine. *Archives of Disease in Childhood,* **62,** 119–122

DEBNEY, L. M. (1984) Visual stimuli as migraine trigger factors. In *Progress in Migraine Research,* vol. 2 (ed. F. C. Rose), Pitman, London, pp. 30–54

DE BRUIJN, J. G., BRUYN, G. W. and KLAWANS, H. L. JR (1976) Further observation on the possible relationship between migraine and serum ammonia levels. *Clinical Neurology and Neurosurgery,* **79,** 151–155

DE CLERCK, F. F. and HERMAN, A. G. (1983) 5-Hydroxytryptamine and platelet aggregation. *Federation Proceedings,* **42,** 228–232

DEL BENE, E. and POGGIONI, M. (1987) Typical and atypical cluster headache in childhood. *Cephalalgia,* Suppl. 6, **7,** 128–130

DEONNA, T. (1978) Troubles neurologiques paroxystiques non épileptiques chez l'enfant. *Revue Medicale de la Suisse Romande,* **98,** 167–175

DEONNA, T. and MARTIN, D. (1981) Benign paroxysmal torticollis in infancy. *Archives of Disease in Childhood,* **56,** 956–959

DEONNA, T., ZIEGLER, A-L. and DESPLAND, P. A. (1984) Paroxysmal visual disturbances of epileptic origin and occipital epilepsy in children. *Neuropediatrics,* **15,** 131–135

DEUBNER, D. C. (1977) An epidemiologic study of migraine and headache in 10–20 year olds. *Headache,* **17,** 173–180

DEVOTO, M., LOZITO, A., STAFFA, G. *et al.* (1986) Segregation analysis of migraine in 128 families. *Cephalalgia,* **6,** 101–105

DEXTER, J. D. and WEITZMAN, E. D. (1970) The relationship of nocturnal headaches to sleep stage patterns. *Neurology,* **20,** 513–518

DITTRICH, J., HAVLOVÁ, M. and NEVŠIMALOVÁ, S. (1979) Paroxysmal hemiparesis in childhood. *Developmental Medicine and Child Neurology,* **21,** 800–807

DOUGLAS, E. F. and WHITE, P. T. (1971) Abdominal epilepsy: a reappraisal. *Journal of Pediatrics,* **78,** 59–67

Drug and Therapeutics Bulletin (1980) Metoclopramide/analgesic combinations for migraine. **18,** (24), 95–96

Drug and Therapeutics Bulletin (1981) Management of migraine. **19,** (18), 69–71

Drug and Therapeutics Bulletin (1987) Migraine and oral contraception. **25,** 95–96

DRUMMOND, P. D. and LANCE, J. W. (1983) Extracranial vascular changes and the source of pain in migraine headache. *Annals of Neurology,* **13,** 32–37

DUNN, D. W. and SNYDER, C. H. (1976) Benign paroxysmal vertigo of childhood. *American Journal of Diseases of Children,* **130,** 1099–1100

DUQUETTE, P., MURRAY, T. J., PLEINES, J. *et al.* (1987) Multiple sclerosis in childhood: clinical profile in 125 patients. *Journal of Pediatrics,* **111,** 359–363

DURKAN, G. P., TROOST, B. T., SLAMOVITS, T. L. *et al.* (1981) Recurrent painless oculomotor palsy in children. A variant of ophthalmoplegic migraine? *Headache,* **21,** 58–62

DVILANSKY, A., RISHPON, S., NATHAN I. *et al.* (1976) Release of platelet 5-hydroxytryptamine by plasma taken from patients during and between migraine attacks. *Pain,* **2,** 315–318

DVORKIN, G. S., ANDERMANN, F., CARPENTER, S. *et al.* (1987) Classical migraine, intractable epilepsy, and multiple strokes: a syndrome related to mitochondrial encephalomyopathy. In *Migraine and Epilepsy* (eds F. Andermann and E. Lugaresi), Butterworths, London pp. 203–232

EBERT, A. G. (1984) Chinese restaurant syndrome. *British Medical Journal,* **289,** 1626

EDMEADS, J. (1985) Towards a pathology of headache. *Headache,* **25,** 117

EDVINSSON, L. (1985) Functional role of perivascular peptides in the control of cerebral circulation. *Trends in Neuroscience,* **8,** 126–131

EDVINSSON, L., FAHREHKRUG, J., HANKO, J. *et al.* (1980) VIP (Vasoactive Intestinal Polypeptide)-containing nerves of intracranial arteries in mammals. *Cell and Tissue Research,* **208,** 135–142

EDVINSSON, L. and UDDMAN, R. (1987) Overview of perivascular neuropeptides in the cerebral circulation. *Cephalalgia,* Suppl. 6, **7,** 269–270

EEG-OLOFSSON, O., ODKVIST, L., LINDSKOG, U. and ANDERSSON, B. (1982) Benign paroxysmal vertigo in childhood. *Acta Otolaryngologica (Stockholm),* **93,** 283–289

EEG-OLOFSSON, O., PETERSEN, I. and SELLDEN, U. (1971) The development of the electroencephalogram in normal children from the age of one through 15 years: paroxysmal activity. *Neuropediatrics,* **2,** 375–404

EGGER, J., CARTER, C. M., WILSON, J. *et al.* (1983) Is migraine food allergy? A double-blind controlled trial of oligoantigenic diet treatment. *Lancet,* **ii,** 865–869

EHYAI, A. and FENICHEL, G. M. (1978) The natural history of acute confusional migraine. *Archives of Neurology,* **35,** 368–369

EMERY, E. S. (1977) Acute confusional state in children with migraine. *Pediatrics,* **60,** 110–114

EPSTEIN, M. T., HOCKADAY, J. M. and HOCKADAY, T. D. R. (1975) Migraine and reproductive hormones throughout the menstrual cycle. *Lancet,* **i,** 543–548

EVIATAR, L. (1981) Vestibular testing in basilar artery migraine. *Annals of Neurology,* **9,** 126–130

EVIATAR, L. and EVIATAR, A. (1977) Vertigo in children: differential diagnosis and treatment. *Pediatrics,* **59,** 833–838

FANCHAMPS, A. (1975) Pharmacodynamic principles of anti-migraine therapy. *Headache,* **15,** 79–90

FARWELL, J. R., DOHRMANN, G. J. and FLANNERY, J. T. (1978) Intracranial neoplasms in infants. *Archives of Neurology,* **35,** 533–537

FEATHERSTONE, H. J. (1985) Migraine and muscle contraction headaches: a continuum. *Headache,* **25,** 194–198

FENICHEL, G. M. (1967) Migraine as a cause of benign paroxysmal vertigo of childhood. *Journal of Pediatrics,* **71,** 114–115

FENICHEL, G. M. (1985) Migraine in children. *Neurologic Clinics,* **3,** 77–94

FENTRESS, D. W., MASEK, B. J., MEHEGAN, J. E. and BENSON, H. (1986) Biofeedback and relaxation response training in the treatment of paediatric migraine. *Developmental Medicine and Child Neurology,* **28,** 139–146

FERRIÈRE, G. (1985) Flunarizine in the prophylactic treatment of pediatric migraine. In *Headache 1985* (Proceedings of the Second International Headache Congress) (eds J. Olesen, P. Tfelt-Hansen, K. Jensen), Copenhagen, pp. 176–177

FITZSIMONS, J. M. (1963) Tuberculous meningitis: a follow up study on 198 cases. *Tubercle,* **44,** 87–102

FITZSIMONS, R. B. and WOLFENDEN, W. H. (1985) Migraine Coma. Meningitic migraine with cerebral oedema associated with a new form of autosomal dominant cerebellar ataxia. *Brain,* **108,** 555–577

FLORES, L. E., WILLIAMS, D. L., BELL, B. A. *et al.* (1986) Delay in the diagnosis of of pediatric brain tumours. *American Journal of Diseases in Children,* **140,** 684–686

FORD, R. P. K. and TAYLOR, B. (1982) Natural history of egg hypersensitivity. *Archives of Disease in Childhood,* **57,** 649–652

FORSYTHE, W. I. (1986) Headache: Part VII – use of sedatives and tranquillizers in the treatment of headaches in adults and children. *International Medicine,* **7,** 169–173

FORSYTHE, W. I., GILLIES, D. and SILLS, M. (1984) Propranolol (Inderal) in the treatment of childhood migraine. *Developmental Medicine and Child Neurology,* **26,** 737–741

FORSYTHE, W. I. and REDMOND, A. (1974) Two controlled trials of tyramine in children with migraine. *Developmental Medicine and Child Neurology,* **16,** 794–799

FOZARD, J. R. (1982) Serotonin, migraine and platelets. *Progress in Pharmacology*, **4/4**, 135–146

FRIEDMAN, A. P., FINLEY, K. H., GRAHAM, J. R. *et al.* (1962a) The classification of headache. *Archives of Neurology*, **6**, 173–176

FRIEDMAN, A. P., HARTER, D. H. and MERRITT, H. H. (1962b) Ophthalmoplegic migraine. *Archives of Neurology*, **7**, 320–327

FRIEDMAN, E. and PAMPIGLIONE, G. (1974) Recurrent headache in children (a clinical and electroencephalographic study). *Archivos de Neurobiologia*, Suppl., **37**, 115–176

FROELICH, W. A., CARTER, C. C., O'LEARY, J. L. and ROSENBAUM, H. E. (1960) Headache in childhood. *Neurology*, **10**, 639–642

GARDNER-MEDWIN, A. R. (1981) Possible roles of vertebrate neuroglia in potassium dynamics, spreading depression and migraine. *Journal of Experimental Biology*, **95**, 111–127

GASCON, G. and BARLOW, C. (1970) Juvenile migraine, presenting as an acute confusional state. *Pediatrics*, **45**, 628–635

GASTAUT, H. (1950) Evidences electrographiques d'un mécanisme sous-cortical dans certaines épilepsies partielles. *Revue Neurologique*, **83**, 396–401

GASTAUT, H. (1982) A new type of epilepsy: benign partial epilepsy of childhood with occipital spike-waves. *Clinical Electroencephalography*, **13**, 13–22

GASTAUT, H. (1985) Benign epilepsy of childhood with occipital paroxysms. In *Epileptic Syndromes in Infancy, Childhood and Adolescence*. (eds J. Roger, C. Dravet, M. Bureau, *et al.*) John Libbey Eurotext, London, pp. 159–170

GATRAD, A. R. (1976) Dystonic reactions to metoclopramide. *Developmental Medicine and Child Neurology*, **18**, 767–769

GAWEL, M., BURKITT, M. and ROSE, F. C. (1979) The platelet release reaction during migraine attacks. *Headache*, **19**, 323–327

GAWEL, M., CONNOLLY, J. F. and ROSE, F. C. (1983) Migraine patients exhibit abnormalities in the visual evoked potential. *Headache*, **23**, 49–52

GEISSINGER, J. D. and BUCY, P. C. (1971) Astrocytomas of the cerebellum in children. *Archives of Neurology*, **24**, 125–135

GELMERS, H. J. (1983) Nimodipine, a new calcium antagonist in the prophylactic treatment of migraine. *Headache*, **23**, 106–109

GENAZZANI, A. R., NAPPI, G., FACCHINETTI, F. *et al.* (1984) Progressive impairment of CSF β-EP levels in migraine sufferers. *Pain*, **18**, 127–133

GHOSE, K., COPPEN, A. and CARROLL, D. (1977) Intravenous tyramine response in migraine before and during treatment with indoramin. *British Medical Journal*, **1**, 1191–1193

GIBBINS, I. L., BRAYDEN, J. E. and BEVAN, J. A. (1984) Distribution and origins of VIP-immunoreactive nerves in the cephalic circulation of the cat. *Peptides*, **5**, 209–212

GILCHRIST, J. M. and COLEMAN, R. A. (1987) Ornithine transcarbamylase deficiency: adult onset of severe symptoms. *Annals of Internal Medicine*, **106**, 556–558

GILLBERG, C. and RASMUSSEN, P. (1982) Abnormal head circumference and learning disability. *Developmental Medicine and Child Neurology*, **24**, 198–199

GILLIES, D., SILLS, M. and FORSYTHE, W. I. (1986) Pizotifen (Sanomigran) in childhood migraine. *European Neurology*, **25**, 32–35

GIROUD, M., D'ATHIS, P., GUARD, O. and DUMAS, R. (1986) Migraine and somnambulism. A survey of 122 migraine patients, *Revue Neurologique*, **142**, 42–46

GLISTA, G. G., MELLINGER, J. F. and ROOKE, E. D. (1975) Familial hemiplegic migraine. *Mayo Clinic Proceedings*, **50**, 307–311

GLOVER, V., LITTLEWOOD, J., SANDLER, M. *et al.* (1983) Biochemical predisposition to dietary migraine: the role of phenolsulphotransferase. *Headache*, **23**, 53–58

GLOVER, V., PEATFIELD, R., ZAMMIT-PACE, R. *et al.* (1981) Platelet monoamine oxidase activity and headache. *Journal of Neurology, Neurosurgery, and Psychiatry*, **44**, 786–790

GLOVER, V., SANDLER, M., GRANT, E. *et al.* (1977) Transitory decrease in platelet monoamine-oxidase activity during migraine attacks. *Lancet*, **i**, 391–393

GOADSBY, P. J., LAMBERT, G. A. and LANCE, J. W. (1986) Stimulation of the trigeminal ganglion increases flow in the extracerebral but not the cerebral circulation of the monkey. *Brain Research*, **381**, 63–67

GOADSBY, P.J. and MACDONALD, G. J. (1985) Extracranial vasodilatation mediated by vasoactive intestinal polypeptide (VIP). *Brain Research*, **329**, 285–288

GOLDEN, G. S. (1979) The Alice in Wonderland syndrome in juvenile migraine. *Pediatrics*, **63**, 517–519

GOLDEN, G. S. and FRENCH, J. H. (1975) Basilar artery migraine in young children. *Pediatrics*, **56**, 722–726

GOLDSTEIN, M. and CHEN, T. C. (1982) The epidemiology of disabling headache. *Advances in Neurology*. **33**, 377–390

GOLLA, F. L. and WINTER, A. L. (1959) Analysis of cerebral response to flicker in patients complaining of episodic headache. *Electroencephalography and Clinical Neurophysiology*, **11**, 539–549

GOLTMAN, A. M. (1936) Mechanism of migraine. *Journal of Allergy*, **7**, 351–355

GOODMAN, L. S. and GILMAN, A. (1970) *Pharmacological Basis of Therapeutics*, 4th edn, MacMillan, New York

GORDON, N. (1977) Normal pressure hydrocephalus and arrested hydrocephalus. *Developmental Medicine and Child Neurology*, **19**, 540–543

GOWERS, W. R. (1907) *The Borderland of Epilepsy*, J & A Churchill, London

GRAFSTEIN, B. (1956) Mechanism of spreading cortical depression. *Journal of Neurophysiology*, **19**, 154–171

GRAHAM, J. R. and WOLFF, H. G. (1938) Mechanism of migraine headache and action of ergotamine tartrate. *Archives of Neurology and Psychiatry*, **39**, 737–763

GRANT, D. N. (1971) Benign intracranial hypertension. *Archives of Disease in Childhood*, **46**, 651–655

GRANT, E. C. G. (1979) Food allergies and migraine. *Lancet*, **i**, 966–969

GREENBLATT, S. H. (1973) Posttraumatic transient cerebral blindness. Association with migraine and seizure diatheses. *Journal of the American Medical Association*, **225**, 1073–1076

GRIFFITH, S. G. and BURNSTOCK, G. (1983) Immunohistochemical demonstration of serotonin in nerves supplying human cerebral and mesenteric blood-vessels. Some speculations about their involvement in vascular disorders. *Lancet*, **i**, 561–562

GRIFFITH, J. H. and DODGE, P. R. (1968) Transient blindness after head injury in children. *New England Journal of Medicine*, **278**, 648–651

GROTEMEYER, K. H., VIAND, R. and BEYKIRCH, K. (1983) Thrombozytenfunktion bei vasomotorischen kopfschmerzen und migränekopfschmerzen. *Deutsche Medizinische Wochenschrift*, **108**, 775–778

GUEST, I. A. and WOOLF, A. L. (1964) Fatal infarction of brain in migraine. *British Medical Journal*, **1**, 225–226

GUIDETTI, V., OTTAVIANO, S., PAGLIARINI, M. *et al.* (1983) Psychological peculiarities in children with recurrent primary headache. *Cephalalgia*, Suppl. 1, **41**, 215–217

GUTHKELCH, A. N. (1977) Benign post-traumatic encephalopathy in young people and its relation to migraine. *Neurosurgery*, **1**, 101–106

HAAS, D. C. and LOURIE, H. (1984) Letter. Delayed deterioration of consciousness after trivial head injury in childhood. *British Medical Journal*, **289**, 1625

HAAS, D. C., PINEDA, G. S. and LOURIE, H. (1975) Juvenile head trauma syndromes and their relationship to migraine. *Archives of Neurology*, **32**, 727–730

HAAS, D. C. and SOVNER, R. D. (1969) Migraine attacks triggered by mild head trauma, and their relation to certain post-traumatic disorders of childhood. *Journal of Neurology, Neurosurgery and Psychiatry*. **32**, 548–554

HACKINSKI, V. C., PORCHAWKA, J. and STEELE, J. C. (1973) Visual symptoms in the migraine syndrome. *Neurology*, **23**, 570–579

HAMMOND, J. (1974) The late sequelae of recurrent vomiting of childhood. *Developmental Medicine and Child Neurology*, **16**, 15–22

HANAKOGLU, A., SOMEKH, E. and FRIED, D. (1984) Benign paroxysmal torticollis in infancy. *Clinical Pediatrics*, **23**, 272–274

HANINGTON, E. (1967) Preliminary report on tyramine headache. *British Medical Journal*, **2**, 550–551

HANINGTON, E. (1974) Monoamine oxidase and migraine. *Lancet*, **ii**, 1148–1149

HANINGTON, E. (1983) Migraine. In *Clinical Reactions to Food* (ed. M. H. Lessof), John Wiley, Chichester, pp. 155–180

HANINGTON, E., JONES, R. J., AMESS, J. A. L. and WACHOWICZ, B. (1981) Migraine: a platelet disorder. *Lancet*, **ii**, 720–723

HARDING, G. F. A., DEBNEY, L. M. and MAHESHWARI, M. (1977) EEG changes associated with hemiplegic migraine in childhood. *Journal of Electrophysiological Technology*, **3**, 90–101

HARE, E. H. (1966) Personal observations on the spectral march of migraine. *Journal of the Neurological Sciences*, **3**, 259–264

HARRISON, M. J. G. (1981) Letter. Hemiplegic migraine. *Journal of Neurology, Neurosurgery and Psychiatry*, **44**, 652–653

HARRISON, R. H. (1975) Psychological testing in headache: a review. *Headache*, **14**, 177–185

HARTLAND, J. (1966) *Medical and Dental Hypnosis and its Clinical Applications*, Baillière, London

HARTLAND, J. (1971) Further observations on the use of 'ego strengthening' techniques. *American Journal of Clinical Hypnosis*, **14**, 1–8

HARVALD, B. and HAUGE, M. (1956) A catamnestic investigation of Danish twins. A preliminary report. *Danish Medical Bulletin*, **3**, 150–158

HASUO, K., TAMURA, S. YASUMORI, K. *et al.* (1987) Computed tomography and angiography in MELAS (mitochondial myopathy, encephalopathy, lactic acidosis and stroke-like episodes); report of 3 cases. *Neuroradiology*, **29**, 393–397

HAWKINS, C. (1979) Food allergies and migraine. *Lancet*, **i**, 1137

HELM, R. M. and FROESE, A. (1981) Binding of the receptors for IgE by various lectins. *International Archives of Allergy and Applied Immunology*, **65**, 81–84

HENDERSON, W. R. and RASKIN, N. H. (1972) 'Hot-dog' headache: individual susceptibility to nitrite. *Lancet*, **ii**, 1162–1163

HENRYK-GUTT, R. and REES, W. L. (1973) Psychological aspects of migraine. *Journal of Psychosomatic Research*, **17**, 141–153

HERBERG, L. J. (1975) The hypothalamus and aminergic pathways in migraine. In *Modern Topics in Migraine* (ed. J. Pearce), William Heinemann Medical, London, pp. 85–95

HERRANZ TANARRO, F. J., SAENZ LOPE, E. and SASSOT, S. C. (1984) La pointe-onde occipitale avec et sans épilepsie bénigne chez l'enfant. *Revue d'Electroencephalographie et de Neurophysiologie Clinique*, **14**, 1–7

HEYCK, H. (1969) Pathogenesis of migraine. *Research and Clinical Studies in Headache*, **2**, 1–28

HEYCK, H. (1973) Varieties of hemiplegic migraine. *Headache*, **12**, 135–142

HILTON-JONES, D. (1988) Venous dural sinus disorders. In *Clinical Neurology* (eds M. Swash and J. Oxbury), Churchill Livingstone, Edinburgh, in press

HINRICHS, W. L. and KEITH, H. M. (1965) Migraine in childhood: follow-up report. *Mayo Clinic Proceedings*, **40**, 593–596

HIRTZ, D. G. and NELSON, K. B. (1985) Cognitive effects of anti-epileptic drugs. In *Recent Advances in Epilepsy*, Vol. 2 (eds T. A. Pedley and B. S. Meldrum), chap. 8, Churchill Livingstone, Edinburgh, pp. 161–181

HOCKADAY, J. M. (1975) Anomalies of carbohydrate metabolism. In *Modern Topics in Migraine* (ed J. Pearce), William Heinemann Medical, London, pp. 124–137

HOCKADAY, J. M. (1978) Late outcome of childhood onset migraine and factors affecting outcome, with particular reference to early and late EEG findings. In *Current Concepts in Migraine Research* (ed. R. Greene), Raven, New York, pp. 41–48

HOCKADAY, J. M. (1979) Basilar migraine in childhood. *Developmental Medicine and Child Neurology*, **21**, 455–463

HOCKADAY, J. M. (1982) Headache in children. *British Journal of Hospital Medicine*, **27**, 383–390

HOCKADAY, J. M. and DEBNEY, L. M. (1988) The EEG in migraine. In *Basic Mechanisms of Headache* (eds. J. Olesen and L. Edvinsson), chap. 32, 365–376, Elsevier, Amsterdam

HOCKADAY, J. M. and ROSE F. C. (1987) A children's migraine clinic. Proceedings of the Third Congress of the International Headache Society, Florence. *Cephalalgia*, Suppl. 6, **7**, 119–121

HOCKADAY, J. M. and WHITTY, C. W. M. (1969) Factors determining the EEG in migraine. *Brain*, **92**, 769–788

HOCKADAY, J. M., WILLIAMSON, D. H. and WHITTY, C. W. M. (1971) Blood glucose levels and fatty acid metabolism in migraine related to fasting. *Lancet*, **i**, 1153–1156

HOLMES, D. S. and BURISH, T. G. (1983) Effectiveness of biofeedback for treating migraine and tension headaches: a review of the evidence. *Journal of Psychosomatic Research*, **27**, 515–532

HOLMES, B., BROGDEN, R. N., HEEL, T. M. and AVERY, G. S. (1984) Flunarizine. A review of its pharmacodynamic and pharmacokinetic properties and therapeutic use. *Drugs,* **27,** 6–44

HOLQUIN, J. and FENICHEL, G. (1967) Migraine. *Journal of Pediatrics,* **70,** 290–297

HONIG, P. J. and CHARNEY, E. B. (1982) Children with brain tumour headaches. *American Journal of Diseases in Children,* **136,** 121–124

HOSKING, G. P., CAVANAGH, N. P. and WILSON, J. (1978) Alternating hemiplegia: complicated migraine of infancy. *Archives of Disease in Childhood,* **53,** 656–659

HUGHES, M., CLARK, N., FORBES, L. and COLIN-JONES, D. G. (1986) A case of scurvy. *British Medical Journal,* **293,** 366

HUGHES, E. C., GOTT, P. S., WEINSTEIN, R. C. and BINGGELI, R. (1985) Migraine: a diagnostic test for etiology of food sensitivity by a nutritionally supported fast and confirmed by long-term report. *Annals of Allergy* **55,** 28–32

HUNGERFORD, G. D., DU BOULAY, G. H. and ZILKHA, K. J. (1976) Computerized axial tomography in patients with severe migraine. *Journal of Neurology, Neurosurgery and Psychiatry,* **39,** 990–994

HUNT, W. E. (1976) Tolosa–Hunt syndrome: one cause of painful ophthalmoplegia. *Journal of Neurosurgery,* **44,** 544–549

HUNT, W. E., MEAGHER, J. N. and LEFEVER, H. E. (1961) Painful ophthalmoplegia: its relation to indolent inflammation of the cavernous sinus. *Neurology,* **11,** 56–62

HURST, W. J. and TOOMEY, P. B. (1981) High performance liquid chromatographic determination of four biogenic amines in chocolate. *Analyst,* **106,** 394–402

IDRISS, Z. H., GUTMAN, L.T. and KRONFOL, N. M. (1978) Brain abscesses in infants and children. Current status of clinical findings, management and prognosis. *Clinical Pediatrics,* **17,** 738–746

ISLER, H., WIESER, H. G. and EGLI, M. (1984) Hemicrania epileptica. In *Progress in Migraine Research 2* (ed. F. C. Rose), Pitman, London,pp. 69–82

JANSEN, I., UDDMAN, R., HOCHERMAN, M. *et al.* (1986) Localization and effects of neuropeptide Y, vasoactive intestinal polypeptide, substance P, and calcitonin gene-related peptide in human temporal arteries. *Annals of Neurology,* **20,** 496–501

JENSEN, K. and OLESEN, J. (1985) Temporal muscle blood flow in common migraine. *Acta Neurologica Scandinavica,* **72,** 561–570

JENSEN, T. S. (1980) Transient global amnesia in childhood. *Developmental Medicine and Child Neurology,* **22,** 654–658

JENSEN, T. S., OLIVARIUS, B. DE F., KRAFT, M. and HANSEN, H. (1981a) Familial hemiplegic migraine. A reappraisal and longterm follow up study. *Cephalalgia,* **1,** 33–39

JENSEN, T. S., VOLDBY, B., OLIVARIUS, B. DE F. and JENSEN F. T. (1981b) Cerebral hemodynamics in familial hemiplegic migraine. *Cephalalgia,* **1,** 121–125

JERRETT, W. A. (1979) Headaches in general practice. *The Practitioner,* **222,** 549–555

JERZMANOWSKI, A. and KLIMEK, A. (1983) Immunoglobulins and complement in migraine. *Cephalalgia,* **3,** 119–123

JESSUP, B. A., NEUFELD, R. W. J. and MERSKEY, H. (1979) Biofeedback therapy for headache and other pain – an evaluative review. *Pain,* **7,** 225–270

JOHNS, D. R. (1986) Migraine provoked by aspartame. *New England Journal of Medicine,* **315,** 456

JONES, V. A. and HUNTER, J. O. (1986) Letter. Pseudo food allergy. *British Medical Journal,* **292,** 623–624

JONKMAN, E. J. and LELIEVELD, M. H. J. (1981) EEG computer analysis in patients with migraine. *Electroencephalography and Clinical Neurophysiology,* **52,** 652–655

JUEL-NIELSEN, N. (1965) Individual and environment. A psychiatric-psychological investigation of monozygotic twins reared apart. *Acta Psychiatrica Scandinavica,* Suppl. 183, **40,** 1–292

KAJDOS, V. (1975) The acupuncture treatment of headache. *American Journal of Acupuncture,* **3,** 34–39

KANDT, R. S. and GOLDSTEIN, G. W. (1985) Steroid-responsive ophthalmoplegia in a child. *Archives of Neurology,* **42,** 589–591

KANDT, R. S. and LEVINE, R. M. (1987) Headache and acute illness in children. *Journal of Child Neurology,* **2,** 22–27

KENNARD, C., GAWEL, M., RUDOLPH, N. DE M. and ROSE, F. C. (1978) Visual evoked potentials in migraine subjects. *Research and Clinical Studies in Headache* **6,** 73–80

KENNEY, R. A. (1986) The Chinese restaurant syndrome: an anecdote revisited. *Food Chemistry and Toxicology,* **24,** 351–354

KESSEL, N. (1979) Reassurance. *Lancet*, **i**, 1128–1133

KINAST, M., LUEDERS, H., ROTHNER, A. D. and ERENBERG, G. (1982) Benign focal epileptic discharges in childhood migraine. *Neurology*, **32**, 1309–1311

KLEE, A. (1968) *A Clinical Study of Migraine with Particular Reference to the Most Severe Cases*, Munksgaard, Copenhagen

KOCH, C. and MELCHIOR, J. C. (1969) Headache in childhood. *Danish Medical Bulletin*, **16**, 109–114

KOEHLER, B. (1980) Benign paroxysmal vertigo of childhood: a migraine equivalent. *European Journal of Pediatrics*, **134**, 149–151

KOENIGSBERGER, M. R., CHUTORIAN, A. M., GOLD, A. P. and SCHVEY, M. S. (1968) Benign paroxysmal vertigo of childhood. *Neurology*, **20**, 1108–1113

KOHLENBERG, R. J. (1982) Tyramine sensitivity in dietary migraine: a critical review. *Headache*, **22**, 30–34

KRÄGELOH, I. and AICARDI, J. (1980) Alternating hemiplegia in infants: report of five cases. *Developmental Medicine and Child Neurology*, **22**, 784–791

KRAUS, D. (1978) Migraine and epilepsy: a case for divorce. *MSc Thesis*, McGill University, Montreal, Canada

KREMENITZER, M. and GOLDEN, G. S. (1974) Letter. Hemiplegic migraine: cerebrospinal fluid abnormalities. *Journal of Pediatrics*, **85**, 139

KRUPP, G. R. and FRIEDMAN, A. P. (1953) Recurrent headache in children: a study of 100 clinic cases. *New York State Journal of Medicine*, **53**, 43–46

KUNKLE, E. C., LUND, D. W. and MAHER, P. J. (1948) Studies on headache. Analysis of vascular mechanisms in headache by use of the human centrifuge, with observations on pain perception under increased positive G. *Archives of Neurology and Psychiatry*, **60**, 253–269

KURTZ, Z., PILLING, D., BLAU, J. N. and PECKHAM, C. (1984) Migraine in children: findings from the National Child Development Study. In *Progress in Migraine Research 2* (ed. F. C. Rose), Pitman, London, pp. 9–17

KUZNIECKY, R. and ROSENBLATT, B. (1987) Benign occipital epilepsy: a family study. *Epilepsia*, **28**, 346–350

LABBE, E. L., WILLIAMSON, D. A. (1984) Treatment of childhood migraine using autogenic feedback training. *Journal of Consulting and Clinical Psychology*, **52**, 968–976

LAGREZE, H. L., TSUDA, Y., HARTMANN, A. and BÜLAU, P. (1986) Effect of flunarizine on regional cerebral blood flow in common and complicated migraine. Pilot study. *European Neurology*, Suppl. 1, **25**, 122–126

LAI, C-W., ZIEGLER, D. K., LANSKY, L. L. and TORRES, F. (1982) Hemiplegic migraine in childhood: Diagnostic and therapeutic aspects. *Journal of Pediatrics*, **101**, 696–699

LAMBERT, G. A., BOGDUK, N., GOADSBY, P. J. et al. (1984) Decreased carotid arterial resistance in cats in response to trigeminal stimulation. *Journal of Neurosurgery*, **61**, 307–315

LANCE, J. W. (1982) *Mechanism and Management of Headache*, 4th edn, Butterworths, London

LANCE, J. W. and ANTHONY, M. (1966) Some clinical aspects of migraine. *Archives of Neurology*, **15**, 356–361

LANCE, J. W., LAMBERT, G. A., GOADSBY, P. J. and DUCKWORTH, J. W. (1983) Brainstem influences on the cephalic circulation: experimental data from cat and monkey of relevance to the mechanism of migraine. *Headache*, **23**, 258–265

Lancet (1980) Leading article. Biofeedback and tension headache. *Lancet*, **ii**, 898–899

Lancet (1982) Leading article. Treatment of migraine. *Lancet*, **i**, 1338–1340

Lancet (1984) Leading article. Headache and depression. *Lancet*, **i**, 495

LANDRIEU, P., EVRARD, P. and LYON, G. (1979) Les convulsions d'origine migraineuse. *Archives Francaises Pédiatrie*, **36**, 498–501

LANZI, G., BALOTTIN, U., GAMBA, N. and FAZZI, E. (1983) Psychological aspects of migraine in childhood. *Cephalalgia*, Suppl. 1, **3**, 218–220

LANZI, G., BALOTTIN, U., BORGATTI, R. et al. (1985) Late post-traumatic headache in pediatric age. *Cephalalgia*, **5**, 211–215

LANZI, G., BALOTTIN, U., FAZZI, E. et al. (1986) Benign paroxysmal vertigo in childhood: a longitudinal study. *Headache*, **26**, 494–497

LAPKIN, M. L., FRENCH, J. H., GOLDEN, G. S. and ROWAN, A. J. (1977) The electroencephalogram in childhood basilar artery migraine. *Neurology*, **27**, 580–583

LAPKIN, M. L. and GOLDEN, G. S. (1978) Basilar artery migraine: a review of 30 cases. *American Journal of Diseases in Children*, **132**, 278–281

LAPLANTE, P., SAINT-HILAIRE, J. M. and BOUVIER, G. (1983) Headache as an epileptic manifestation. *Neurology*, **33**, 1493–1495

LAURITZEN, M. (1985) On the possible relation of spreading cortical depression to classical migraine. *Cephalalgia*, Suppl. 2, **5**, 47–51

LAURITZEN, M. (1986) Spreading cortical depression as a mechanism of the aura in classic migraine. In *The Prelude to the Migraine Attack* (ed. W. K. Amery and A. Wauquier), Baillière Tindall, London, pp. 134–141

LAURITZEN, M. (1987) Cortical spreading depression as a putative migraine mechanism. *Trends in Neurosciences*, **10**, 8–13

LAURITZEN, M. and OLESEN, J. (1984) Regional cerebral blood flow during migraine attacks by Xenon-133 inhalation and emission tomography. *Brain*, **107**, 447–461

LEÃO, A. A. P. (1944) Spreading depression of activity in the cerebral cortex. *Journal of Neurophysiology*, **7**, 359–390

LEÃO, A. A. P. (1986) What is cortical spreading depression? In *The Prelude to the Migraine Attack* (ed. W. K. Amery and A Wauquier), Baillière Tindall, London, pp. 129–133

LECHNER, H., OTT, E., FAZEKAS, F. and PILGER, E. (1985) Evidence of enhanced platelet aggregation and platelet sensitivity in migraine patients. *Cephalalgia*, Suppl. 2, **5**, 89–91

LEE, C. H. and LANCE, J. W. (1977) Migraine stupor. *Headache*, **17**, 32–38

LEES, F. (1962) The migrainous symptoms of cerebral angiomata. *Journal of Neurology, Neurosurgery and Psychiatry*, **25**, 45–50

LEES, F. and WATKINS, S. M. (1963) Loss of consciousness in migraine. *Lancet*, **ii**, 647–650

LENHARD, L. and WAITE, P. M. (1983) Acupuncture in the prophylactic treatment of migraine headaches: pilot study. *New Zealand Medical Journal*, **96**, 663–666

LENNOX, W. G. and LENNOX, M. A. (1960) Borderlands of epilepsy. In *Epilepsy and Related Disorders*, Little, Brown, Boston

LESSOF, M. H., WRAITH, D. G., MERRETT, T. G. *et al.* (1980) Food allergy and intolerance in 100 patients – local and systemic effects. *Quarterly Journal of Medicine (New Series)* **49**, 259–271

LEVIN, S. (1982) Moya-Moya disease. *Developmental Medicine and Child Neurology*, **24**, 850–853

LEVITON, A. (1984) To what extent does food sensitivity contribute to headache recurrence? *Developmental Medicine and Child Neurology*, **26**, 542–545

LEVITON, A. (1986) Do learning handicaps and headache cluster? *Journal of Child Neurology*, **1**, 372–377

LEVITON, A., SLACK, W. V., MASEK, B. *et al.* (1984a) A computerized behavioral assessment for children with headaches. *Headache*, **24**, 182–185

LEVITON, A., SLACK, W. V., BANA, D. and GRAHAM, J. R. (1984b) Age-related headache characteristics. *Archives of Neurology*, **41**, 762–764

LEWIS, E. G., DUSTAMN, R. E. and BECK, E. C. (1972) Evoked response similarity in monozygotic, dizygotic and unrelated individuals: comparative study. *Electroencephalography and Clinical Neurophysiology*, **32**, 309–316

LING, W., OFTEDAL, G. and WEINBERG, W. (1970) Depressive illness in childhood presenting as severe headache. *American Journal of Diseases of Children*, **120**, 122–124

LINET, M. S. and STEWART, W. F. (1984) Migraine headache: epidemiologic perspectives. *Epidemiologic Reviews*, **6**, 107–139

LIPPMAN, C. W. (1952) Certain hallucinations peculiar to migraine. *Journal of Nervous and Mental Disease*, **116**, 346–351

LIPSON, E. H. and ROBERTSON, W. C. Jr (1978) Paroxysmal torticollis of infancy: familial occurence. *American Journal of Diseases of Children*, **132**, 422–423

LIPTON, S. A. (1986) Prevention of classic migraine headache by digital massage of the superficial temporal arteries during visual aura. *Annals of Neurology*, **19**, 515–516

LITTLEWOOD, J. T., GIBB, C., GLOVER, V. *et al.* (1988) Red wine as a cause of migraine. *Lancet*, **i**, 558–559

LITTLEWOOD, J., GLOVER, V., SANDLER, M. *et al.* (1982) Platelet phenolsulphotransferase deficiency in dietary migraine. *Lancet*, **i**, 983–986

LITTLEWOOD, J. T., GLOVER, V. and SANDLER, M. (1987) Red wine contains a potent inhibitor of phenolsulphotransferase. *British Journal of Clinical Pharmacology*, **19**, 275–278

LIVEING, E. (1873) *On Megrim, Sick-headache and Some Allied Disorders: A Contribution to the Pathology of Nerve Storms*, Churchill, London

LLOYD, J. K. and SCRIVER, C. R. (eds) (1985) *Genetic and Metabolic Disease in Pediatrics*, Butterworths, London

LOEHLIN, J. C. (1982) Are personality traits differentially heritable? *Behaviour Genetics*, **12**, 417–428

LOH, L., NATHAN, P. W., SCHOTT, G. D. and ZILKHA, K. J. (1984) Acupuncture versus medical treatment for migraine and muscle tension headaches. *Journal of Neurology, Neurosurgery and Psychiatry*, **47**, 333–337

LOMBROSO, C. T. and LERMAN, P. (1967) Breath-holding spells (cyanotic and pallid infantile syncope). *Pediatrics*, **39**, 563–581

LORD, G. D. A. and DUCKWORTH, J. W. (1978) Complement and immune complex studies in migraine. *Headache*, **18**, 255–260

LOUIS, P. (1981) A double-blind placebo-controlled prophylactic study of flunarizine (Sibelium) in migraine. *Headache*, **21**, 235–239

LOUIS, P. and SPIERINGS, E. L. H. (1982) Comparison of flunarizine (Sibelium) and pizotifen (Sanomigran) in migraine treatment: a double-blind study. *Cephalalgia*, **2**, 197–203

LUCAS, R. N. (1977) Migraine in twins. *Journal of Psychosomatic Research*, **20**, 147–156

LUDVIGSSON, J. (1974) Propranolol used in prophylaxis of migraine in children. *Acta Neurologica Scandinavica*, **50**, 109–115

LUNDBERG, P. O. (1975) Abdominal migraine: diagnosis and therapy. *Headache*, **15**, 122–125

MCCANN, J. (1982) Migraines may manifest as vertigo (news). *Journal of the American Medical Association*, **247**, 956–957

MACDONALD, A. and FORSYTHE, W. I. (1986) The cost of nutrition and diet therapy for low-income families. *Human Nutrition*, **40A**, 87–96

MACDONALD, A., FORSYTHE, W. I. and MINFORD, A. M. B. (1987) Practical problems associated with the dietary management of migraine. In *Current Problems in Neurology: 4. Advances in Headache Research* (Proceedings of the Sixth International Migraine Symposium) (ed. F. C. Rose), John Libbey, London, pp. 113–116

MCGRATH, P. J., GOODMAN, J. T., FIRESTONE, P. et al. (1983) Recurrent abdominal pain: a psychogenic disorder? *Archives of Disease in Childhood*, **58**, 888–890

MACKENZIE, I. (1953) The clinical presentation of the cerebral angioma: a review of 50 cases. *Brain*, **76**, 184–214

MAGNI, G., PIERRI, M. and DONZELLI, F. (1987) Recurrent abdominal in children: a long term follow up. *European Journal of Pediatrics*, **146**, 72–74

MAKI, Y., NAKADA, Y., NOSE, T. and YOSHII, Y. (1976) Clinical and radioisotopic follow-up study of 'Moya-Moya'. *Child's Brain*, **2**, 257–271

MALETZKY, B. M., KLOTTER, J. (1976) Addiction to diazepam. *International Journal of Addiction*, **11**, 95–115

MANSFIELD, J. (1986) *The Migraine Revolution. The New Drug-free Solution*. Thorsons Publishing Group, Wellingborough, pp. 119–120

MANSFIELD, L. E., VAUGHAN, T. R., WALLER, S. F. et al. (1985) Food allergy and adult migraine: double-blind and mediator confirmation of an allergic etiology. *Annals of Allergy*, **55**, 126–129

MARATOS, J. and WILKINSON, M. (1982) Migraine in children: a medical and psychiatric study. *Cephalalgia*, **2**, 179–187

MARCUSSEN, R. M. and WOLFF, H. G. (1950) Studies on headache; effects of carbon dioxide – oxygen mixtures given during preheadache phase of the migraine attack; further analysis of the pain mechanisms in headache. *Archives of Neurology and Psychiatry*, **63**, 42–51

MARTIN, P. R. and MATHEWS, A. M. (1978) Tension headaches: psychophysiological investigation and treatment. *Journal of Psychosomatic Research*, **22**, 389–399

MASYCZEK, R. and OUGH, C. S. (1983) The 'red wine reaction' syndrome. *American Journal of Enology and Viticulture*, **34**, 260–264

MATHEW, N. T., MEYER, J. S., WELCH, K. M. A. and NEBLETT, C. R. (1977) Abnormal CT scans in migraine. *Headache*, **16**, 272–279

MATSON, D. D. (1965) Intracranial arterial aneurysms in childhood. *Journal of Neurosurgery*, **23**, 578–583

MATTHEWS, W. B. (1972) Footballer's migraine. *British Medical Journal*, **2**, 326–327

MAYBERG, M., LANGER, R. S., ZERVAS, N. T. and MOSKOWITZ, M. A. (1981) Perivascular meningeal projections from cat trigeminal ganglia: possible pathway for vascular headaches in man. *Science*, **213**, 228–230

MEDINA, J. L. and DIAMOND, S. (1976) Migraine and atopy. *Headache*, **15**, 271–274

MEDINA, J. L. and DIAMOND, S. (1978) The role of diet in migraine. *Headache*, **18**, 31–34

MENKEN, M. (1978) Transient confusion after minor head injury. *Clinical Pediatrics*, **17**, 421–422

MENKES, J. H. (1985) *Textbook of Child Neurology*, 3rd edn, Lea Febiger, Philadelphia, p. 309

MENT, L. R., DUNCAN, C. C., PARCELLS, P. R. and COLLINS, W. F. (1980) Evaluation of complicated migraine in childhood. *Child's Brain*, **7**, 261–266

MERRETT, T. G., GAWEL, M. J. and PEATFIELD, R. C. (1980) Food allergy in migraine. *Lancet*, **ii**, 532

MERRETT, J., PEATFIELD, R. C., ROSE, F. C. and MERRETT, T. G. (1983) Food related antibodies in headache patients. *Journal of Neurology, Neurosurgery, and Psychiatry*, **46**, 738–742

METTINGER, K. L. and ERICSON, K. (1982) Fibromuscular dysplasia and the brain. I: Observations on angiographic, clinical and genetic characteristics. *Stroke*, **13**, 46–52

MEYER, J. S. (1985) Calcium channel blockers in the prophylactic treatment of vascular headaches. *Annals of Internal Medicine*, **102**, 395–397

MEYER, J. S. and HARDENBERG, J. (1983) Clinical effectiveness of calcium entry blockers in the prophylactic treatment of migraine and cluster headaches. *Headache*, **23**, 266–277

MILITERNI, R., TRIPODI, D., ARGENZIO, G. and QUINTO, A. M. (1983) Il torticollo parossistico nell' infanzia. *Pediatria (Napoli)*, **91**, 265–267

MILLER, F. J. W., COURT, S. D. M., KNOX, E. G. and BRANDON, S. (1974) *The School Years in Newcastle Upon Tyne 1952–62: being a further contribution to the study of a thousand families*, Oxford University Press, Oxford, p. 280

MILLICHAP, J. G. (1978) Recurrent headaches in 100 children. *Child's Brain*, **4**, 95–105

MILLICHAP, J. G., LOMBROSO, C. T. and LENNOX, W. G. (1955) Cyclic vomiting as a form of epilepsy in children. *Pediatrics*, **15**, 705–714

MINFORD, A. M. B., MACDONALD, A. and LITTLEWOOD, J. M. (1982) Food intolerance and food allergy in children: a review of 68 cases. *Archives of Disease in Childhood*, **57**, 742–747

MIRA, E., PIACENTINO, G., LANZI, G. and BALOTTIN, U. (1984) Benign paroxysmal vertigo in childhood. Diagnostic significance of vestibular examination and headache provocation tests. *Acta Otolaryngologica Supplement*, **406**, 271–274

MITCHELL, R. (1967) Migraine in childhood. *Developmental Medicine and Child Neurology*, **9**, 641–643

MOFFETT, A., SWASH, M. and SCOTT, D. F. (1972) Effect of tyramine in migraine: a double-blind study. *Journal of Neurology, Neurosurgery, and Psychiatry*, **35**, 496–499

MOFFETT, A. M., SWASH, M. and SCOTT, D. F. (1974) Effect of chocolate in migraine: a double-blind study. *Journal of Neurology, Neurosurgery, and Psychiatry*, **37**, 445–448

MONAGHAN, J. and DODGE, J. A. (1980) The role of stressful life events in childhood recurrent abdominal pain. In *Proceedings of the Fifty-Second Annual Meeting of the British Paediatric Association York*, British Paediatric Association, p. 55

MONERET-VAUTRIN, D. A. (1983) False food allergies: non-specific reactions to foodstuffs. In *Clinical Reactions to Food* (ed. M. H. Lessof), John Wiley, Chichester, pp. 135–153

MONRO, J., BROSTOFF, J., CARINI, C. and ZILKHA, K. (1980) Food allergy in migraine. *Lancet*, **ii**, 1–4

MONRO, J., CARINI, C. and BROSTOFF, J. (1984) Migraine is a food-allergic disease. *Lancet*, **ii**, 719–721

MOORE, T. L., RYAN, R. E., POHL, D. A. *et al.* (1980) Immunoglobulin, complement, and immune complex levels during a migraine attack. *Headache*, **20**, 9–12

MORI, K., MIWA, S., MURATA, T. *et al.* (1979) Basilar artery occlusion in childhood. *Archives of Neurology*, **36**, 100–102

MOSKOWITZ, M. A. (1984) The neurobiology of vascular head pain. *Annals of Neurology*, **16**, 157–168

MOSKOWITZ, M. A., BREZINA, L. R. and KUO, C. (1986) Dynorphin B-containing perivascular axons and sensory neurotransmitter mechanisms in brain blood vessels. *Cephalalgia*, **6**, 81–86

MOSS, G. and WATERS, W. E. (1974) Headache and migraine in a girls' grammar school. In *The Epidemiology of Migraine* (ed. W. E. Waters), Boehringer, Ingelheim, pp. 49–58

MÜCK-SELER, D., DEANOVIC, Z. and DUPELJ, M. (1979) Platelet serotonin (5-HT) and 5-HT releasing factor in plasma of migrainous patients. *Headache*, **19**, 14–17

MÜLLER, D and MÜLLER, J. (1977) Die familiäre hemiplegische Migräne. *Zeitschrift für Arztliche Fortbildung (Jena)*, **71**, 763–767

NATTERO, G., LISINO, F., BRANDI, G. *et al.* (1976) Reserpine for migraine prophylaxis. *Headache*, **15**, 270–281

NAUGHTEN, E., NEWTON, R. WEINDLING, A. M. and BOWER, B. D. (1981) Tuberculous meningitis in children. *Lancet*, **ii**, 973–975

NEW, P. F. J. and SCOTT, W. R. (1975) *Computed Tomography of the Brain and Orbit – EMI Scanning*, Williams and Wilkins, Baltimore, pp. 359–361

NEWTON, R. and AICARDI, J. (1983) Clinical findings in children with occipital spike-waves suppressed by eye-opening. *Neurology*, **33**, 1526–1529

NICOL, A. R. (1982) Psychogenic abdominal pain in children. *British Journal of Hospital Medicine*, **27**, 351–353

NIMMO, J., HEADING, R. C., TOTHILL, P. and PRESCOTT, L. F. (1973) Pharmacological modifying of gastric emptying: effects of propantheline and metoclopramide on paracetamol absorption. *British Medical Journal*, **1**, 587–589

NORONHA, M. J. (1985) Double-blind randomised cross-over trial of timolol in migraine prophylaxis in children. In *Headache 1985* (Proceedings of the Second International Headache Congress), (eds J. Olesen, P. Tfelt-Hansen, K. Jensen), Copenhagen, pp. 174–175

NORREGAARD, T. V. and MOSKOWITZ, M. A. (1985) Substance P and the sensory innervation of intracranial and extracranial feline cephalic arteries. *Brain*, **108**, 517–533

NOVAK, G. P. and MOSHE, S. L. (1985) Brainstem glioma presenting as paroxysmal headache. *Developmental Medicine and Child Neurology*, **27**, 379–382

NUECHTERLEIN, K. H. and HOLROYD, J. C. (1980) Biofeedback in the treatment of tension headache. Current status. *Archives of General Psychiatry*, **37**, 866–873

O'CONNOR, T. P. and VAN DER KOOY, D. (1986) Pattern of intracranial and extracranial projections of trigeminal ganglion cells, *Journal of Neuroscience*, **6**, 2200–2207

O'DONNELL, B. (1985) *Abdominal Pain in Children*, Blackwell Scientific, Oxford

O'DONOHOE, N. V. (1971) Annotation. Abdominal epilepsy. *Developmental Medicine and Child Neurology*, **13**, 798–814

OGUNYEMI, A. O. (1984) Prevalence of headache among Nigerian university students. *Headache*, **24**, 127–130

OKA, H., KAKO, M., MATUSUSHIMA, M. and ANDO, K. (1977) Traumatic spreading depression syndrome. Review of a particular type of head injury in 37 patients. *Brain*, **100**, 287–298

OLESEN, J. (1985) Migraine and regional cerebral blood flow. *Trends in Neurosciences*, **8**, 318–321

OLESEN, J. (1986) The Pathophysiology of migraine. In *Headache* (eds P. J. Vinken, G. W. Bruyn, H. L. Klawans and F. C. Rose), *Handbook of Clinical Neurology*, **48**, chap. 6, 59–83, Elsevier, Amsterdam

OLESEN, J., AEBELHOLT, A. and VEILIS, B. (1979) The Copenhagen Acute Headache Clinic: organisation, patient material and treatment results. *Headache*, **19**, 223–227

OLESEN, J. and EDVINSSON, L. (EDS). (1988) *Basic Mechanisms of Headache*, Elsevier, Amsterdam

OLESEN, J., TFELT-HANSEN, P., HENRIKSEN, L. and LARSEN, B. (1981) The common migraine attack may not be initiated by cerebral ischaemia. *Lancet*, **ii**, 438–440

OLIVARIUS, B. DE F. and JENSEN, T. S. (1979) Transient global amnesia in migraine. *Headache*, **19**, 335–338

OLNESS, K., MACDONALD, J. T. and UDEN, D. L. (1987) Comparison of self-hypnosis and propranolol in the treatment of juvenile classic migraine. *Pediatrics*, **79**, 593–597

OSTER, J. (1972) Recurrent abdominal pain, headache and limb pains in children and adolescents. *Pediatrics*, **50**, 429–436

OSTFELD, A. M., REIS, D. J., GOODELL, H. and WOLFF, H. G. (1955) Headache and hydration: the significance of two varieties of fluid accumulation in patients with vascular headache of the migraine type. *Archives of Internal Medicine*, **96**, 142–152

PANAYIOTOPOULOS, C. P. (1980) Basilar migraine, seizures, and severe epileptic EEG abnormalities. *Neurology*, **30**, 1122–1125

PANAYIOTOPOULOS, C. P. (1981) Inhibitory effect of central vision on occipital lobe seizures. *Neurology*, **31**, 1330–1333

PANDEY, G. N., DORUS, E., SHAUGHNESSY, R. and DAVIS, J. M. (1979) Genetic control of platelet monoamine oxidase activity: studies on normal families. *Life Sciences*, **25**, 1173–1178

PARAIN, D. and SAMSON-DOLLFUS, D. (1984) Electroencephalograms in basilar artery migraine. *Electroencephalography and Clinical Neurophysiology*, **58**, 392–399

PARKES, J. D. (1975) Relief of pain: headache, facial neuralgia, migraine and phantom limb. *British Medical Journal*, **4**, 90–92

PARRINO, L., PIETRINI, V., SPAGGIARI, C. and TERZANO, M. G. (1986) Acute confusional migraine attacks resolved by sleep: lack of significant abnormalities in post-ictal polysomnograms. *Cephalalgia*, **6**, 95–100

PARSONAGE, M. (1975) Electroencephalographic studies in migraine. In *Modern Topics in Migraine* (ed. J. Pearce), William Heinemann Medical, London, pp. 72–84

PASSCHIER, J. and ORLEBEKE, J. F. (1985) Headaches and stress in schoolchildren: an epidemiological study. *Cephalalgia*, **5**, 167–176

PATEL, A. N. and RICHARDSON, A. E. (1971) Ruptured intracranial aneurysms in first two decades of life; study of 58 patients. *Journal of Neurosurgery*, **35**, 571–576

PAULIN, J. M., WAAL-MANNING, H. J, SIMPSON, F. O. and KNIGHT, R. G. (1985) The prevalence of headache in a small New Zealand town. *Headache*, **25**, 147–151

PAVLAKIS, S. G., PHILLIPS, P. C., DIMAURO, S. *et al.* (1984) Mitochondrial myopathy, encephalopathy, lactic acidosis, and stroke like episodes: a distinctive clinical syndrome. *Annals of Neurology*, **16**, 481–488

PEARCE, J. M. S. (1971) Insulin induced hypoglycaemia in migraine. *Journal of Neurology, Neurosurgery, and Psychiatry*, **34**, 154–156

PEARCE, J. M. S. (1984a) Migraine: a cerebral disorder. *Lancet*, **ii**, 86–89

PEARCE, J. M. S. (1984b) Letter. Food allergy and migraine. *Lancet*, **ii**, 926

PEARCE, J. M. S. (1985) Is migraine explained by Leao's spreading depression? *Lancet*, **ii**, 763–766

PEARCE, J. M. S. and FOSTER, J. B. (1965) An investigation of complicated migraine. *Neurology*, **15**, 333–340

PEARSON, D. J. (1985) Food allergy, hypersensitivity and intolerance. *Journal of the Royal College of Physicians of London*, **19**, 154–162

PEARSON, D. J., RIX, K. J. B. and BENTLEY, S. J. (1983) Food allergy: how much in the mind? A clinical and psychiatric study of suspected food hypersensitivity. *Lancet*, **i**, 1259–1261

PEATFIELD, R. C. (1986) *Headache* (series eds J. P. Conomy and M. Swash) *Clinical Medicine and the Nervous System*, Springer, London

PEATFIELD, R. C., GLOVER, V., LITTLEWOOD, J. M. *et al.* (1984) The prevalence of diet-induced migraine. *Cephalalgia*, **4**, 179–183

PEATFIELD, R. C., PETTY, R. G. and ROSE, F. C. (1983) Double-blind comparison of mefenamic acid and acetaminophen (paracetamol) in migraine. *Cephalalgia*, **3**, 129–134

PECKHAM, C. and BUTLER, N. (1978) National study of asthma in children. *Journal of Epidemiology and Community Health*, **32**, 79–85

PEROUTKA, S. J. and ALLEN, G. S. (1984) The calcium antagonist properties of cyproheptadine: implications for antimigraine action. *Neurology (New York)*, **34**, 304–309

PERRY, T. L., HANSEN, S., HESTRIN, M. and MACINTYRE, L. (1965) Exogenous urinary amines of plant origin. *Clinica Chimica Acta*, **11**, 24–34

PETTY, R. K. H., HARDING, A. E. and MORGAN-HUGHES, J. A. (1986) The clinical features of mitochondrial myopathy. *Brain*, **109**, 915–938

PIETRINI, V., TERZANO, M. G., D'ANDREA, G. *et al.* (1987) Acute confusional migraine: clinical and electroencephalographic aspects. *Cephalalgia*, **7**, 29–37

PIKOFF, H. (1984) Is the muscular model of headache still viable? A review of conflicting data. *Headache*, **24**, 186–198

PIPILI, E. and POYSER, N. L. (1981) Effects of nerve stimulation and of administration of noradrenaline or potassium chloride upon the release of prostaglandins I_2, E_2. and $F_2\alpha$ from the perfused mesenteric arterial bed of the rabbit. *British Journal of Pharmacology*, **72**, 89–93

PLANT, G. T. (1986) The fortification spectra of migraine. *British Medical Journal*, **293**, 1613–1617

PRADALIER, A., LAUNAY, J. M., DRY, J. and DREUX, C. (1983a) Rôle de la sérotonine plaquettaire dans la migraine commune. *La Presse Médicale*, **12**, 2311–2314

PRADALIER, A., WEINMAN, S., LAUNAY, J. M. *et al.* (1983b) Total IgE, Specific IgE, and prick-tests against foods in common migraine – a prospective study. *Cephalalgia*, **3**, 231–234

PRENSKY, A. L. (1976) Migraine and migrainous variants in pediatric patients. *Pediatric Clinics of North America*, **23**, 461–471

PRENSKY, A. L. and SOMMER, D. (1979) Diagnosis and treatment of migraine in children. *Neurology*, **29**, 506–510

PUCA, F., MINERVINI, M. G., GENCO, S. *et al.* (1985) EEG spectral analysis in common and classic migraine. In *Headache 1985* (Proceedings of the Second International Headache Congress) (eds J. Olesen, P. Tfelt-Hansen, K. Jensen), Copenhagen, pp. 382–383

RAAB, E. L. and SNYDER, C. H. (1970) Letters. Paroxysmal torticollis in infancy. *American Journal of Disease in Children*, **119**, 378

RASCOL, A., MONTASTRUC, J. L. and RASCOL, O. (1986) Flunarizine versus pizotifen: a double-blind study in the prophylaxis of migraine. *Headache*, **26**, 83–85

RASKIN, N. H. (1981) Chemical headaches. *Annual Reviews of Medicine*, **32**, 63–71

RASKIN, N. H. and APPENZELLER, O. (1980) *Headache. Major Problems in Internal Medicine*, **19**, Saunders, Philadelphia

REGISTRAR-GENERAL'S ANNUAL REPORT (1985) Mortality Statistics. Office of Population Censuses and Surveys England and Wales, Mortality Statistics Childhood 1985, HMSO, London

REINHART, J. B., EVANS, S. L. and MCFADDEN, D. L. (1977) Cyclic vomiting in children: seen through the psychiatrist's eye. *Pediatrics*, **59**, 371–377

RIGG, C. A. (1975) Migraine in children and adolescents. *Acta Paediatrica Scandinavica*, Suppl 256, 19–24

RITZ, A., JACOBI, G. and EMRICH, R. (1981) Komplizierte Migräne beim Kind. *Monatsschrift für Kinderheilkunde*, **129**, 504–512

RIX, K. J. B., PEARSON, D. J. and BENTLEY, S. J. (1984) A psychiatric study of patients with supposed food allergy *British Journal of Psychiatry*, **145**, 121–126

ROBERTON, W. C. and SCHNITZLER, E. R. (1978) Ophthalmoplegic migraine in infancy. *Pediatrics*, **61**, 886–888

ROBERTS, M. H. T. (1984) 5-Hydroxytryptamine and antinociception. *Neuropharmacology*, **23**, 1529–1536

ROBERTSON, D. M., BARBOR, P. and HULL, D. (1982) Unusual injury? Recent injury in normal children and children with suspected non-accidental injury *British Medical Journal*, **285**, 1399–1401

ROSSI, L. N., MUMENTHALER, M. and VASSELLA, F. (1980) Complicated migraine (migraine accompagnée) in children. *Neuropediatrics*, **11**, 27–35

ROSSI, L. N., VASELLA, F., BAJC, O., *et al.* (1985) Benign migraine-like syndrome with CSF pleocytosis in children. *Developmental Medicine and Child Neurology*, **27**, 192–198

ROTH, J. A. (1986) Sulfoconjugation: role in neurotransmitter and secretory protein activity. *Trends in Pharmacological Sciences*, **7**, 404–407

ROTHNER, A. D., ERENBERG, G. CRUSE, R. P., *et al.* (1982) Acute aphasic migraine. *Headache*, **22**, 150–151 (Abstract)

ROWE, P. C., NEWMAN, S. L. and BRUSILOW, S. W. (1986) Natural history of symptomatic partial ornithine transcarbamylase deficiency. *New England Journal of Medicine*, **314**, 541–547

ROYAL COLLEGE OF PHYSICIANS AND THE BRITISH NUTRITION FOUNDATION (1984) Food intolerance and food aversion. *Journal of the Royal College of Physicians of London*, **18**, 83–123

RUSH, J. A. (1983) Pseudotumour cerebri. *British Journal of Hospital Medicine*, **29**, 320–325

RUSHTON, J. G. and ROOKE, E. D. (1962) Brain tumor headache. *Headache*, **2**, 147–152

RUSSELL, A. (1973) The implications of hyperammonemia in rare and common disorders, including migraine. *Mount Sinai Journal of Medicine*, **40**, 609–630

RYAN, R. E. JR. (1974) A clinical study of tyramine as an aetiological factor in migraine. A double-blind study. *Headache*, **14**, 43–48

RYAN, R. E. SR., DIAMOND, S., RYAN, R. E. JR. (1975) Double-blind study of clonidine and placebo for the prophylactic treatment of migraine *Headache*, **15**, 202–210

SACHS, H., SEVILLA, F., BARBERIS, P., *et al.* (1985) Headache in the rural village of Quiroga, Ecuador. *Headache*, **25**, 109–193

SACKS, O. W. (1970) *Migraine. The Evolution of a Common Disorder*, Faber and Faber, London

SACQUEGNA, T., CORTELLI, P., BALDRATI, A., et al. (1985) Impairment of consciousness in migraine. In Headache 1985 (Proceedings of the Second International Headache Congress) (eds J. Olesen, P. Tfelt-Hansen, K. Jensen), Copenhagen, pp. 334–335

SALFIELD, S. A. W., WARDLEY, B. L., HOULSBY, W. T., et al. (1987) Controlled study of exclusion of dietary vasoactive amines in migraine. Archives of Disease in Childhood, 62, 458–460

SALMON, M. A. (1977) Migraine in childhood. Nursing Mirror, 145, 16–17

SALMON, M. A. (1983) Diagnosis of abdominal migraine in children. In Migraine in Childhood (ed. J. Wilson), The Medicine Publishing Foundation, Oxford, pp. 1–2

SALMON, M. A. (1985) Abdominal migraine in childhood and its place in the evolution of adult (cranial) migraine. In Headache 1985 (Proceedings of the Second International Headache Congress) (eds J. Olesen, P. Tfelt-Hansen, K. Jensen), Copenhagen, p. 182

SALMON, M. A. and WALTERS, D. D. (1985) Letter. Pizotifen in the prophylaxis of cyclical vomiting. Lancet, i, 1036–1037

SANDLER, M., YOUDIM, M. B. H. and HANINGTON, E. (1974) A phenylethylamine oxidising defect in migraine. Nature, 250, 335–337

SANDLER, M., YOUDIM, M. B. H., SOUTHGATE, J. and HANINGTON, E. (1970) The role of tyramine in migraine: some possible biochemical mechanisms. In Background to Migraine (Third Migraine Symposium, 1969) (ed. A. L. Cochrane), William Heinemann Medical Books, London, pp. 103–112

SANNER, G. and BERGSTRÖM, B. (1979) Benign paroxysmal torticollis in infancy. Acta Paediatrica Scandinavica, 68, 219–223

SANTUCCI, M., CORTELLI, P., ROSSI, P. G., et al. (1986) L-5-Hydroxytryptophan versus placebo in childhood migraine prophylaxis: a double-blind cross-over study. Cephalalgia, 6, 155–157

SANTUCCI, M., ROSSI, P. G., AMBROSETTO, G., et al. (1985) Migraine and benign epilepsy with Rolandic spikes in childhood. Developmental Medicine and Child Neurology, 27, 60–62

SAPER, J. R. (ed.) (1983) Headache Disorders: Current Concepts and Treatment Strategies, Wright, Bristol

SAPER, J. R. and JONES, J. M. (1986) Ergotamine tartrate dependency: features and possible mechanisms. Clinical Neuropharmacology, 9, 244–256

SARGENT, J. D., GREEN, E. E. and WALTERS, E. D. (1973) Preliminary report on the use of autogenic feedback training in the treatment of migraine and tension headaches. Psychosomatic Medicine, 35, 129–135

SCHADÉ, J. P. (1959) Maturational aspects of EEG and of spreading depression in rabbit. Journal of Neurophysiology, 22, 245–257

SCHEPANK, H. (1974) Erg- and eltfaktorem bei Neurosen. Teifenpsychologische Untersuchungen an 50 Zwillingspaaren, Springer-Verlag, Berlin,

SCHOENEN, J., JAMART, B. and DELWAIDE, P. J. (1987) Topographic EEG mapping in common and classic migraine during and between attacks. In Current Problems in Neurology: 4. Advances in Headache Research (Proceedings of the Sixth International Migraine Symposium) (ed. F. C. Rose), John Libbey, London, pp. 25–33

SCHULTE, F. J. (1984) Intracranial tumours in childhood: concepts of treatment and prognosis Neuropediatrics, 15, 3–12

SCHWEITZER, J. W., FRIEDHOFF, A. J. and SCHWARTZ, R. (1975) Chocolate, β-phenylethylamine and migraine re-examined. Nature (London) 257, 256

SEDZIMER, C. B. and ROBINSON, J. (1973) Intracranial haemorrhage in children and adolescents. Journal of Neurosurgery, 38, 269–281

SELBY, G. and LANCE, J. W. (1960) Observations on 500 cases of migraine and allied vascular headache. Journal of Neurology, Neurosurgery and Psychiatry, 23, 23–32

SESHIA, S. S., REGGIN, J. D. and STANWICK, R. S. (1985) Migraine and complex seizures in children. Epilepsia, 26, 232–236

SETHI, T. J., LESSOF, M. H., KEMENY, D. M., et al. (1987) How reliable are commercial allergy tests? Lancet, i, 92–94

SHAW, S. W. J., JOHNSON, R. H. and KEOGH, H. J. (1978) Oral tyramine in dietary migraine sufferers. In Current Concepts in Migraine Research (ed. R. Greene), Raven, New York, pp. 31–39

SICUTERI, F., BUFFONI, F., ANSELMI, B. and DEL BIANCO, P. L. (1972) An enzyme (MAO) defect on the platelet in migraine. *Research and Clinical Studies in Headache*, **3**, 245–251

SILLANPÄÄ, M. (1976) Prevalence of migraine and other headache in Finnish children starting school. *Headache*, **15**, 288–290

SILLANPÄÄ, M. (1983a) Changes in the prevalence of migraine and other headaches during the first seven school years. *Headache*, **23**, 15–19

SILLANPÄÄ, M. (1983b) Prevalence of headache in prepuberty. *Headache*, **23**, 10–14

SILLANPÄÄ, M. and PIEKKALA, P. (1984) Prevalence of migraine and other headaches in early puberty. *Scandinavian Journal of Primary Health Care*, **2**, 27–32

SILLS, M., CONGDON, P. and FORSYTHE, W. I. (1982) Clonidine and childhood migraine – a pilot and double-blind study. *Developmental Medicine and Child Neurology*, **24**, 837–841

SJAASTAD, O. (1980) So-called 'tension headache': a term in need of revision? *Current Medical Research and Opinion*, Suppl 9, **6**, 41–54

SLATTER, K. H. (1968) Some clinical and EEG findings in patients with migraine. *Brain*, **91**, 85–98

SMALL, P. and WATERS, W. E. (1974) Headache and migraine in a comprehensive school. In *The Epidemiology of Migraine* (ed. W. E. Waters), Boehringer, Ingelheim, pp. 59–67

SMITH, I., KELLOW, A. H., MULLEN, P. E. and HANINGTON, E. (1971) Dietary migraine and tyramine metabolism. *Nature*, **230**, 246–248

SMITH, K. D. (1981) Abnormal head circumference in learning disabled children. *Developmental Medicine and Child Neurology*, **23**, 626–632

SMYTH, V. O. G. and WINTER, A. L. (1964) The EEG in migraine. *Electroencephalography and Clinical Neurophysiology*, **16**, 194–202

SNOEK, J. W., MINDERHOUD, J. M. and WILMINK, J. T. (1984) Delayed deterioration following mild head injury in children. *Brain*, **107**, 15–36

SNYDER, C. H. (1969) Paroxysmal torticollis in infancy. A possible form of labyrinthitis. *American Journal of Diseases in Children*, **117**, 458–460

SOLIMAN, H., PRADALIER, A., LAUNAY, J-M., et al. (1987) Decreased phenol and tyramine sulphoconjugation by platelets in dietary migraine. In *Current Problems in Neurology: 4. Advances in Headache Research* (Proceedings of the Sixth International Migraine Symposium) (ed. F. C. Rose), John Libbey, London, pp. 117–121

SORGE, F. and MARANO, E. (1985) Flunarizine v. placebo in childhood migraine. A double-blind study. *Cephalalgia*, Suppl. 2, **5**, 145–148

SOVAK, M., KUNZEL, M., DALESSIO, D. J. and LANG, J. H. (1980) C-1 inhibitor levels in migraineurs and normals. *Headache*, **20**, 132–133

SPACCAVENTO, L. J. and SOLOMON, G. D. (1984) Migraine as an etiology of stroke in young adults. *Headache*, **24**, 19–22

SPARKS, J. P. (1978) The incidence of migraine in schoolchildren. *The Practitioner*, **221**, 407–411

STENSRUD, P. and SJAASTAD, O. (1980) Comparative trial of Tenormin (atenolol) and Inderal (propranolol) in migraine. *Headache*, **20**, 204–207

STEPHENSON, J. B. P. (1978) Reflex anoxic seizures ('white breath-holding'): nonepileptic vagal attacks. *Archives of Disease in Childhood*, **53**, 193–200

STICKLER, G. B. and MURPHY, D. B. (1979) Recurrent abdominal pain. *American Journal of Diseases of Children*, **133**, 486–489

STILL, J. L. and COTTOM, D. (1967) Severe hypertension in childhood. *Archives of Disease in Childhood*, **42**, 34–39

STONE, R. T. and BARBERO, G. J. (1970) Recurrent abdominal pain in childhood. *Pediatrics*, **45**, 732–738

STURZENEGGER, M. N. and MEIENBERG, O. (1985) Basilar artery migraine: A follow-up study of 82 cases. *Headache*, **25**, 408–415

SWAIMAN, K. F. and FRANK, Y. (1978) Seizure headaches in children. *Developmental Medicine and Child Neurology*, **20**, 580–585

SWANSON, J. W. and VICK, N. A. (1978) Basilar artery migraine. *Neurology*, **28**, 782–786

SWARTZ, M. N. and DODGE, P. R. (1965) Bacterial meningitis. A review of selected aspects. *New England Journal of Medicine*, **272**, 725–731, 779–787

SYMON, D. N. K. and RUSSELL, G. (1986) Abdominal migraine: a childhood syndrome defined. *Cephalalgia*, **6**, 223–228

TAL, Y., DUNN, H. G. and CHRICHTON, J. U. (1984) Childhood migraine – a dangerous diagnosis? *Acta Paediatrica Scandinavica*, **73**, 55–59

TER BERG, H. W. M., BIJLSMA, J. B. and WILLEMSE, J. (1987) Familial occurrence of intracranial aneurysms in childhood: a case report and review of the literature. *Neuropediatrics*, **18**, 227–230

TERRENCE, C. F. and SAMAHA, F. J. (1973) The Tolosa-Hunt syndrome (painful ophthalmoplegia) in children. *Developmental Medicine and Child Neurology*, **15**, 506–509

TERZANO, M. G., MANZONI, G. C. and PARRINO, L. (1987) Benign epilepsy with occipital paroxysms and migraine: the question of intercalated attacks In *Migraine and Epilepsy* (eds F. Andermann and E. Lugaresi), Butterworths, Londo.., pp. 83–96

TFELT-HANSEN, P. and KRABBE, A. A. (1981) Ergotamine abuse. Do patients benefit from withdrawal? *Cephalalgia*, **1**, 29–32

TFELT-HANSEN, P., OLESEN, J., AEBELHOLT- KRABBE, A., *et al.* (1980) A double-blind study of metoclopramide in the treatment of migraine attacks. *Journal of Neurology, Neurosurgery and Psychiatry*, **43**, 369–371

THOMPSON, R. A. and BIRD, A. G. (1983) How necessary are specific IgE antibody tests in allergy diagnosis? *Lancet*, **i**, 169–172

THOMPSON, R. A. and PRIɔ .AM, H. F. (1969) Infantile cerebral aneurysm associated with ophthalmoplegia and quadriparesis. *N urology*, **19**, 785–789

THONNARD-NEUMANN, E. and NECKERS, L. M. (1981) T-Lymphocytes in migraine. *Annals of Allergy*, **47**, 325–327

THRUSH, D. (1984) Does ergotamine work for migraine? In *Dilemmas in the Management of the Neurological Patient* (eds. C. Warlow and J. Garfield), chap. 10, Churchill Livingstone, Edinburgh, pp. 106–114

TINUPER, P., CORTELLI, P., SACQUEGNA, T. and LUGARESI, E. (1985) Classic migraine attack complicated by confusional state – EEG and CT study. *Cephalalgia*, **5**, 63–68

TODD, J. (1955) Syndrome of Alice in Wonderland. *Canadian Medical Association Journal*, **73**, 701–704

TOKOLA, R. and HOKKANEN, E. (1978) Propranolol for acute migraine. *British Medical Journal*, **2**, 1089

TROOST, B. T., MARK, L. E. and MAROON, J. C. (1979) Resolution of classic migraine after removal of an occipital lobe arterio-venous malformation. *Annals of Neurology*, **5**, 199–201

TRUED, S. (1974) Migraine in childhood. *Journal of the American Medical Women's Association*, **29**, 78–83

TUNIS, M. M. and WOLFF, H. G. (1953) Studies on headache; long-term observations of reactivity of cranial arteries in subjects with vascular headache of migraine type. *Archives of Neurology and Psychiatry*, **70**, 551–557

UNGE, G., MALMGREN, R., OLSSON, P., *et al.* (1983) Effects of dietary protein-tryptophan restriction upon 5-HT uptake by platelets and clinical symptoms in migraine-like headache. *Cephalalgia*, **3**, 213–218

UNGER, A. H. and UNGER, L. (1952) Migraine is an allergic disease. *Journal of Allergy*, **23**, 429–440

VAHLQUIST, B. (1955) Migraine in children. *International Archives of Allergy*, **7**, 348–352

VAHLQUIST, B. and HACKZELL, G. (1949) Migraine of early onset. *Acta Paediatrica*, **38**, 622–636

VAN BUREN, J. M. (1963) The abdominal aura. A study of abdominal sensations occurring in epilepsy and produced by depth stimulation. *Electroencephalography and Clinical Neurophysiology*, **15**, 1–19

VAN PELT, W. and ANDERMANN, F. (1964) On the early onset of ophthalmoplegic migraine. *American Journal of Diseases of Children*, **107**, 628–631

VERCELLETTO, P., CLER, J. M. and FRIOL, M. (1979) Vertiges et migraine basilaire. Place nosologique des vertiges Benins de l'enfant. *Revue d'Otoneuro-ophtalmologie*, **51**, 231–238

VERRET, S. and STEELE, J. C. (1971) Alternating hemiplegia in childhood: a report of eight patients with complicated migraine beginning in infancy. *Pediatrics*, **47**, 675–680

VIJAYAN, N., GOULD, S. and WATSON, C. (1980) Exposure to sun and precipitation of migraine. *Headache*, **20**, 42–43

VISINTINI, D., TRABATTONI, G., MANZONI, G. C., *et al.* (1986) Immunological studies in cluster headache and migraine. *Headache*, **26**, 398–402

VOLANS, G. N. (1975) The effect of metoclopramide on the absorption of effervescent aspirin in migraine. *British Journal of Clinical Pharmacology*, **2**, 57–63

WAINSCOTT, G., KASPI, T. and VOLANS, G. N. (1976) The influence of thiethylperazine on the absorption of effervescent aspirin in migraine. *British Journal of Clinical Pharmacology*, **3**, 1015–1021

WALSER, H. and ISLER, H. (1982) Frontal intermittent rhythmic delta activity, impairment of consciousness and migraine. *Headache,* **22,** 74–80

WALSH, F. B. and HOYT, W. F. (1969) *Clinical Neuro-Ophthalmology,* 3rd edn, Wilkins and Wilkins, Baltimore

WALSH, J. P. and O'DOHERTY, D. S. (1960) A possible explanation of the mechanism of ophthalmoplegic migraine. *Neurology,* **10,** 1079–1084

WATERS, W. E. (1971) Migraine: intelligence, social class and familial prevalence. *British Medical Journal,* **2,** 77–81

WATERS, W. E. (1972) Migraine and symptoms in childhood: bilious attacks, travel sickness and eczema. *Headache,* **12,** 55–61

WATERS, W. E. (1973) The epidemiological enigma of migraine. *International Journal of Epidemiology,* **2,** 189–194

WATERS, W. E. (ed.) (1974a) *The Epidemiology of Migraine. Six Surveys of Headache and Migraine,* Boehringer-Ingelheim, Bracknell

WATERS, W. E. (ed.) (1974b) Surveys of headache and migraine: conclusions. In *The Epidemiology of Migraine. Six Surveys of Headache and Migraine,* Boehringer-Ingelheim, Bracknell, pp. 68–76

WATERS, W. E. (1986) *Headache,* Croom Helm, London

WATSON, P. and STEELE, J. C. (1974) Paroxysmal dysequilibrium in the migraine syndrome of childhood. *Archives of Otolaryngology,* **99,** 177–179

WEERASURIYA, K., PATEL, I. and TURNER, P. (1982) Beta-adrenoceptor blockade and migraine. *Cephalalgia,* **2,** 33–45

WERCH, S. C. (1964) Letter. Allergy to propionates. *Journal of the American Medical Association,* **187,** 872

WERDER, D. S. and SARGENT, J. D. (1984) A study of childhood headache ‡using biofeedback as a treatment alternative. *Headache,* **24,** 122–126

WERLIN, S. L., D'SOUZA, B. J., HOGAN, W. J., et al. (1980) Sandifer syndrome. *Developmental Medicine and Child Neurology,* **22,** 374–378

WHITTY, C. W. M. (1953) Familial hemiplegic migraine. *Journal of Neurology Neurosurgery and Psychiatry,* **16,** 172–177

WHITTY, C. W. M. (1967) Migraine without headache. *Lancet,* **ii,** 283–285

WHITTY, C. W. M. (1972) Leading article. Migraine and epilepsy. *Hemicrania,* **4,** 2–4

WHITTY, C. W. M. (1986) Familial hemiplegic migraine. In *Headache* (eds. P. J. Vinken, G. W. Bruyn, H. L. Klawans and F. C. Rose), *Handbook of Clinical Neurology,* **48,** chap. 11, 141–153, Elsevier, Amsterdam

WHITTY, C. M. and HOCKADAY, J. M. (1968) Migraine: a follow-up study of 92 patients. *British Medical Journal,* **1,** 735–736

WHITTY, C. W. M., HOCKADAY, J. M. and WHITTY, M. M. (1966) The effect of oral contraceptives on migraine. *Lancet,* **i,** 856–859

WILKINS, A., NIMMO-SMITH, I., TAIT, A., et al. (1984) A neurological basis for visual discomfort. *Brain,* **107,** 989–1017

WILKINSON, M. (1984) Adverse reactions to drugs used in the treatment of migraine. *Adverse Drug Reaction Bulletin,* no. 108, October

WILKINSON, M. (1986) Clinical features of migraine. In *Headache* (eds. P. J. Vinken, G. W. Bruyn and H. L. Klawans and F. C. Rose), *Handbook of Clinical Neurology,* **48,** chap. 9, 117–133, Elsevier, Amsterdam

WILKINSON, M., WILLIAMS, K. and LEYTON, M. (1978) Observations on the treatment of an acute attack of migraine. *Research and Clinical Studies in Headache,* **6,** 141–146

WONG, G., KNUCKEY, N. W. and GUBBAY, S. S. (1983) Subarachnoid haemorrhage in children caused by cerebral tumour. *Journal of Neurology, Neurosurgery and Psychiatry,* **46,** 449–450

WOODY, R. C. and BLAW, M. E. (1986) Ophthalmoplegic migraine in infancy. *Clinical Pediatrics,* **25,** 82–84

WORLD FEDERATION OF NEUROLOGY RESEARCH GROUP ON MIGRAINE AND HEADACHE (1969) Meeting of the Research group on Migraine and Headache. *Journal of the Neurological Sciences,* **9,** 202

YAMAMOTO, M. and MEYER, J. S. (1980) Hemicranial disorder of vasomotor adrenoceptors in migraine and cluster headache. *Headache,* **20,** 321–325

YOUDIM, M. B. H., CARTER, S. B., SANDLER, M., *et al.* (1971) Conjugation defect in tyramine-sensitive migraine. *Nature,* **230,** 127–128

YOUNG, G. B. and BLUME, W. T. (1983) Painful epileptic seizures. *Brain,* **106,** 537–554

ZIEGLER, D. K. (1978) The epidemiology and genetics of migraine. *Research and Clinical Studies in Headache,* **5,** 21–33

ZIEGLER, D. K. (1979) Headache syndromes: problems of definition. *Psychosomatics,* **20,** 443–447

ZIEGLER, D. K. (1984) Clinical and familial characteristics of patients with classical migraine. In *Progress in Migraine Research,* vol. 2 (ed. F. C. Rose), Pitman, London, pp.1–8

ZIEGLER, D. K., HASSANEIN, R. and HASSANEIN, K. (1972) Headache syndromes suggested by factor analysis of symptom variables in a headache prone population. *Journal of Chronic Diseases,* **25,** 353–363

ZIEGLER, D. K., HASSANEIN, R. S., HARRIS, D. and STEWART, R. (1975) Headache in a non-clinic twin population. *Headache,* **14,** 213–218

ZIEGLER, D. K. and STEWART, R. A. (1977) Failure of tyramine to induce migraine. *Neurology,* **27,** 725–726

ZIEGLER, D. K. and WONG, G. (1967) Migraine in childhood: clinical and EEG study of families. *Epilepsia,* **8,** 171–187

Index